Behind My Stethoscope

Letters of Solidarity, Encouragement, and Advice to
New and Seasoned Nurses

Kim R. Edwards RN

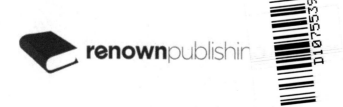

Renown Publishing
www.renownpublishing.com

Behind My Stethoscope / Kim R. Edwards
ISBN-13: 978-1-952602-15-3

With over forty years of nursing experience, I find it hard to pick one or even a few people to dedicate this book to. The love, support, lessons, discipline, and advice came from a lot of places. There has been equal time between home family and work family, and I've learned things from everyone I've come in contact with. There is no way to mention them all, but there are a few people who need a special thanks:

Mama—for believing that I could do anything.

Megan—for just being you and for understanding the life of having a mama as a nurse (you had lots of experience).

Big Meg—for always answering and being on the other end of the phone, laughing and having some sort of answer.

Terrie—for giving me the courage to step out and do it.

Auntie M—for the variety of roles you have played through the years.

And last but not least, my niece, Kasey—who gave me the reason for writing this book. I am so proud of you and the nurse that you are, and I can't wait to watch your career. You've got this, girl!

To the rest of you who know me, have worked with me, were my patients, and have been my friends: thanks to all of you. This book would not have been possible if not for the role that each of you has played in my life.

CONTENTS

Dear Kasey

Over forty years. That's how long I have been in the world of nursing. Four years at a nursing home. Four years of nursing school and one year as a working nursing extern. One year as a GRN (graduate registered nurse waiting to find out if I passed the boards or not), five years in Neuro ICU, and eleven years in an outpatient unit. Nine years in the Recovery Room, two years in wound care, and the last three years as a bedside nurse on an outpatient unit. All at the same hospital.

It's time. After being in some form of nursing for over forty years, I'm turning in my stethoscope. It isn't because I'm tired of nursing, because I got fired, or because I'm too old (I'm a very young 58). It's just because I'm done. But I wouldn't change my experiences, and I don't regret my decision to spend all those years working as a nurse. I've poured my heart and soul into my career, but I'm ready for the next chapter.

I began this book about my nursing experience to provide you and other new nurses with information that just can't be learned in school. Over the course of my career, my titles were as follows: nurse's aide, student nurse, nurse extern, graduate nurse, registered nurse, assistant nurse manager, nurse manager, and clinical nurse.

I can't tell you that it was my life calling or that I'm the world's most compassionate person, but I cared very much about my patients and the staff I supervised. Overall, I enjoyed my job. But nursing is hard—not learning the science of it, but the actual doing-it-ever-day part.

In school, you learn how to make beds and give shots and enemas. You learn sterilization techniques for putting in Foleys and tubes and for doing dressing changes. And let's not forget about all the drugs. You'll learn about drugs you cannot even pronounce. You'll learn what they are for and how to make sure the right amount has been ordered for the right reason, and you'll continue learning about them your entire career. Hopefully, someone will make the names easier to pronounce so your patient has a chance of remembering the name instead of just telling you they take "a little pink pill" for their blood pressure.

You learn to perform complete assessments—recognizing heart rhythms, lung sounds, and those very noisy bowel sounds. You learn to recognize signs and symptoms for every disease and condition known to mankind. During your nursing career, there will be new diseases. You'll see advances in the way we provide care to our patients, and the development of new technology will be beyond amazing.

Continuing Education

There is a lot that happens before you ever take your first step as a nurse. You pick your nursing school, you pass your boards, you get hired, and then you eagerly and nervously start your nursing career. And what happens after that is truly amazing and terrifying: *you're* responsible for the care of another person. Your patients need you in so many ways, and no one can really prepare you for that. You have to experience it for yourself.

Some things will never change, no matter what's discovered or developed. As a nurse, you'll cry with your patients and laugh with your patients. And yes, I can assure you that you'll experience *every* emotion in between. You'll meet and care for people and families from all walks of life and will walk a portion of their journey with them. You'll affect their lives, and believe me, they will affect yours. Rich and poor, young and old, happy and sad, blessed and lonely—they will cross your path for a while, and you'll be forever changed by each one you meet. For good or bad, you'll leave a mark on them as well.

I had the honor and privilege of working with so many amazing people who taught me countless lessons. In my opinion, some of the best nursing teams have *nothing* to do with the initials behind their names. I recognize that some people went to school, worked hard, paid a lot of money, and have earned their initials. But being a good nurse has more to do with heart and intention. The best nursing team is the team with the best people on it. The secret isn't in their title; it's in who they are as people, what they know, and how much respect you show them for their experience.

I can put you in a classroom all day every day, but putting that first nasogastric tube down a real patient, rather than a simulator, is different. It'll be different every time for the rest of your career, and you'll learn tricks about what works, what doesn't work, and what won't ever work (even if that's what the textbook or policy says). Real-life experiences count, in some ways even more than school. Don't get me wrong—we need schooling. But the learning doesn't stop when we graduate or when we leave formal school.

As the need for bedside nurses increases, the need for instructors also increases. We need everyone who can help us learn to better care for patients *at the bedside*: unit secretaries, EKG techs, nurse techs, nurse's aides, nursing students, LPNs, RNs, BSNs, and MSNs.

No Pressure

I know exactly how you feel being a newbie. I was there. I don't care how old I am—I remember what it was like being a student nurse and a new nurse. It's not readily forgotten. You're learning to save lives, and that's not an easy job. You have so much to remember, and so many things get in the way—the family, the patients themselves, and even your own nerves.

You're working with a complete team, but as the RN on the team, the full responsibility falls on you. You have to make sure the doctor orders the right medications, at the right dose, for the right patient, and ensure that it's administered at the right intervals. You're relying on their skills, and relying on the pharmacist to get it right. You have computers to help you with some of the steps, but the last person to push that medication into the patient is *you*. And you better make sure it's the right one. No pressure.

You're with the patient way more than any other health professional. Physical therapy, occupational therapy, respiratory therapy, dietary, and countless other people come into that room sporadically. But as the nurse, you are there the most.

We Can't Fix It

Nurses are sometimes seen as angels by patients or family members who have experienced a hospital stay. Other times, they feel we don't care the way we should, or that we could be doing better. In the end, we are all human. Although I always tried to give everything I had to my patients, sometimes it still wasn't enough, and for that, I'm sorry. I've laughed and cried in the room with my patients and families, and I've left the room to quietly shed tears or get my emotions together.

As a nurse, you're often times seeing people at a difficult time in their life, maybe the most difficult season they've ever experienced. For the majority of my career, I worked with people who needed surgery—something either was broken or had to be removed. Maybe the person needed a biopsy for a cancer diagnosis.

People who are in the hospital *don't want to be there*, and all the compassion in the world won't help them cope with horrible news.

It took me a long time to finally understand there was nothing I could do to make it better—to change their situation or ease their suffering. Yes, I could hold their hand, listen to whatever they needed to talk about, get them pain medicine, help them call their family and friends, or simply sit in the room with them while they cried. But I couldn't fix it, and you won't be able to fix it, either. Sometimes that reality is emotionally draining, but it's also a precious gift. You get to meet people right where they are in the middle of their hardest days. And while you can't change their circumstances, you get to *be with* them and offer care and support. It is not an easy career, and it might be one of the most thankless jobs ever—but what you're doing *matters*.

Over the years, I've heard people complain about the care they received. As nurses, we don't always get it right, but we certainly try. The good nurses outweigh the bad—most of us genuinely care about the patients and their outcomes. In fact, a "bad nurse" is often just one who reached their limit in a sometimes-traumatic field of work.

Room after room after room, we walk in and everyone is sick. Some are getting better, some are getting worse, and some don't know what their future holds. We work long hours, often putting in overtime to stay late and help out. Sometimes we are helping the other nurses or spending time checking on a patient whose time is running out and whose family hasn't arrived yet. She doesn't want to die alone, and I don't want her to die alone, so I slip back in after my shift to sit at her bedside, hoping whatever time I can stay will make a difference.

We all get frustrated by the amount of work we have to

do, by not taking a break, by the long work hours that keeps us from our families. Some nurses are so close to burnout that they lash out at others.

In my forty years working with one particular nurse, I never heard her make a single complaint or inappropriate comment to patients, families, or coworkers. However, that nurse had an on-the-job heart attack, which I believe came from keeping so much inside. Hopefully, my advice to new nurses can help them avoid burning out or leaving nursing altogether.

Every day that I went to work, I intended to make a positive difference in someone's life, aiming never to cause any additional strain, pain, or worry. And every day, I hoped that would be enough.

Thank You

I've always known that as a nurse, I was caring for the patient *and* their family. Everyone I've cared for touched me in some way and helped me learn life lessons—sometimes the easy way, sometimes the hard way. I'd like to thank all of them for touching my life in a way that helped make nursing such a wonderful and rewarding career.

To my patients, thank you for your time; to my patients' families, thank you for allowing me to care for your family member; and to my fellow nurses, thank you for always being there, even when it got really hard.

You've Got This

Nursing is an amazing career. This book will discuss

my experience with all aspects of nursing, including the range of emotions I felt. The privacy and confidentiality of my patients and their families have always been, and continue to be, one of my primary concerns. Details in the stories have been changed so no one will be able to identify who my patients were. The stories are only meant to provide insight and encouragement for those just starting out in the field. You are in for adventure and life-changing experiences! If I can do anything to help prepare you for your career and help you give better care to your patients, I'm all in.

While some of my experiences will come across as funny, this isn't meant in any way to be disrespectful to any of my patients or their families.

As you read about my experiences, I hope you'll realize all you can do is your best—even on days when it feels like your best isn't good enough. I will tell you things I wish someone had told me at the beginning of my career.

I also hope this book helps you see things from a slightly different perspective than what you learned in nursing school. Nursing school helps lay the foundation, but after you pass your boards, you'll start your own unique nursing experience. The purpose of this book is to give newer nurses some insights into nursing and hopefully lead experienced nurses to smile or recall parts of their own careers. It isn't "the Nursing Bible"; it isn't the way things should be done; and it's certainly not the only way. Sometimes I will tell you how I did things the wrong way.

Though each person's nursing career will be unique to them, I want to do for you what I wish someone had done for me: talk to you, nurse to nurse, about the realities of the career that lies ahead of you.

My stories may make you smile or cry, be angry or frustrated, laugh or be grossed out—just like every day you spend as a nurse. I simply hope they make you feel something—anything—because if nothing else, a career in nursing is full of emotions. You *never* know what will happen, and each day is different. Life as a nurse is *never* dull or boring.

Kasey, you're the pilot, and your career is the plane. You're on the runway, ready to take off and fly. Your plane is full. There are a lot of people on it to help you, and everyone is depending on you. You have co-pilots and stewards (RNs, PCAs, unit secretaries). You have passengers (patients, families, and doctors), people in the air traffic control center (supervisors, nurse directors), and people throughout the airport helping you get the passengers on and off the airplane and to their destination. Even though you're a great pilot and can do a lot, you can't do it by yourself. You have a lot to learn, controls to watch, and thousands of other things to do.

But don't worry—because *you've got this.*

Love,
Aunt Kim

CHAPTER ONE

Forever Changed

Dear Kasey,

In some ways, my years as a nurse's aide at a nursing home taught me more than I ever learned in the hospital setting. Maybe it was because I took care of the same patients every day. That job was an opportunity to learn so many life lessons. But being a kid at the time, I didn't realize it until much later. Everyone you work with, team members or patients, will teach you something. You just have to be open to learning it.

Love, Aunt Kim

Death is just as much a part of life as birth is. Maybe more. I spent four summers working in a wonderful nursing home as a nurse's aide. I learned so much about life and death, not just from a professional standpoint but from a personal one as well. When we come into this world, we seemingly know nothing; when we die, we all hope we have learned some lessons and gained knowledge along the way.

I was sixteen years old and very "wet behind the ears."

We had four wings of patients with twenty patients per wing. Forty years later, I can still tell you the names of *all* my patients on my assigned wing. I remember their faces as if they were my own family.

These are a few memories of them:

One patient wouldn't leave her room for breakfast down the hall unless her jewelry was on.

Another had clothes that she only wore on specific days of the week.

If the military man started talking, you needed to sit down and listen. He was a history book, and it was amazing.

The two sets of couples could teach you a lot if you just watched their interactions. They had each been married for over sixty years, and however they accomplished that, it was amazing.

What can I say about the lady, over one hundred years old, who wasn't supposed to be off the floor but who would somehow figure out how to run away to get her piece of bread, no matter how many times we brought her back? For me, it was the right thing to do to "be busy" and not realize she was gone. She always came back. Living for over a century had earned her some rights in my book.

The purple lady had all the money in the world, yet it couldn't make her happy. I've often thought about what it would be like to win the lottery, but seeing her so rich and so unhappy helped me learn early on that money certainly can't buy you everything.

As I think back to those summers, I realize I learned many life lessons working with and caring for those patients.

Four important events coincided with my four summers there:

1. I became great friends with an aide who would eventually go to school to be a nurse. She had a husband and young son. Her husband didn't want her to go to school, so he threw her books out into the rain and hid her car keys. But she wanted to be a nurse more than anything, so she kept after it. I did my best to encourage and support her career goals. I even helped her dry her books out. We spent many days laughing and talking about life and all the things we planned to do.

She was *never* late to work, but one foggy morning she didn't show up. The charge nurse and I knew something was wrong. We later found out that on the way to work, she and another car had run a stop sign at the same time. The other car clipped her in the right, back bumper and slammed her into a telephone pole. She was fine, but the seat belt was locked, and she couldn't get out. The guy who had hit her was trying to help her out when the car blew up. She didn't survive.

I never understood why someone so young—with a child and with such great plans and so much love to give to future patients—had to die in such an awful way.

2. I experienced the loss of my own grannie. She was very sick. Here I was facing the end of life with patients her age, but not once did I realize I could lose her, too.

3. I decided to become a nurse. I had worked with patients for so long that it eventually made sense to go to nursing school. Prior to that, I had always wanted to be a

veterinarian and never thought about being a nurse. But after four summers at the nursing home, it seemed the obvious answer.

4. The last summer at the nursing home, I met a coworker who was attending school at FSU. She talked me into applying, I got in, and as they say, the rest is history.

Looking back now, I know I was in that place for a reason. As you go through your career, you'll work with patients and their families and have a myriad of experiences—good and bad, happy and sad. And one day, you'll realize you experienced all those things for a reason and learned many valuable lessons through it all.

CHAPTER TWO

Why I Chose Nursing

Dear Kasey,

When I first started out in nursing, I had no plans, thoughts, or ideas as to what my future looked like. I had a good job, I had job security, and I could do it. What I didn't know was that in becoming a nurse, I had changed the very basics of who I was. As a nurse, you can't ever put it away. If a family member is having a health problem, they will call and ask your advice. When you're at the mall and you see someone having trouble breathing, you'll assess them to see what's going on. And God forbid that someone actually goes down in front of you. You'll be on them, assessing, directing people as to what to do, and you'll take care of that patient until the paramedics get there. You'll never be able to not be a nurse. It's in your soul. And that's a good thing.

There are as many different reasons why people went to school to be a nurse as there are nurses. It doesn't matter how or why you got here—you're here. Welcome to our world. This is the story of how I ended up in nursing school.

Love, Aunt Kim

What was I thinking? Why in the world did I choose nursing as a career? The truth of the matter is, I really didn't choose nursing; it sorta kinda picked me. I grew up on a farm and dreamed of being a vet. But do you know how long veterinarians have to go to school? I wanted (and needed) a career where I could get through school in a relatively short period of time and support myself with the salary.

I went for my Associate of Science (A.S.) degree at a community college within an hour of where I grew up. It was a huge adjustment for this little country girl. While I was getting my A.S. degree, my roommate got her RN. I somehow realized that by going to the University of Florida (UF) or Florida State University (FSU) for my nursing degree, I could finish in 2.5 years with a Bachelor of Science in Nursing (BSN) rather than just an RN.

Now, before anyone jumps, I have no issue with an RN versus a BSN. As a nurse manager, I thought two-year RN students were better prepared clinical-wise than many four-year students. But everything else being equal, I'd hire an experienced BSN over an experienced RN because the RN would probably go back to school to get her BSN, so she would need time off from work.

Please don't beat me up for this. Being a good nurse doesn't depend on the type of degree you have. One of the best preceptor nurses (an experienced nurse you temporarily get paired with, who teaches/shows you how to do certain procedures) I ever had in my career was a licensed practical nurse (LPN). She was so knowledgeable, friendly, patient, and experienced, and a great teacher able to articulate things well. All her patients loved her. She was incredible.

As a nurse's aide, I worked with LPNs in the nursing

home, and they had an amazing level of experience and knowledge. I had a lot of great preceptors and role models as nurses, ranging from nurse's aides to Chief Nursing Officers. It's who you are and how you treat your patients, families, coworkers, and staff that tell people what kind of nurse you are.

So back to *why* I picked nursing. After the two-year degree, when I applied to FSU and UF, I got accepted to both. I needed one semester of prerequisites, and if I passed, I could enter their nursing program and finish up in two years. That sounded great.

Now, here's a part of the story that's a little sad but kind of cool in the end. My grannie was so excited about me going to nursing school. She knew I had applied and that we were waiting for the results. I had only applied to FSU and UF. I was hoping to go to UF because I grew up a Gator fan, but the FSU acceptance letter came in first. My grannie was so proud. She knew I wanted to go to UF, but at least I had been accepted to FSU and would be going to nursing school. Though I was happy that she was happy, I still planned to see if I could get into UF.

My grannie had bad heart problems. Up to this point, she'd already had four heart attacks and was a diabetic. That weekend, she died. The next week, my acceptance letter to UF came in. I didn't even have to think about it: my grannie had known that I could go to nursing school at FSU, so with both acceptance letters in hand, I chose FSU—because that's where my grannie thought I was going.

I won't get into which school is better. I won't do a "Go 'Noles!" chant or a rousing round of the Gator fight song. *My grannie thought I would attend FSU when she died, so that's where I went. End of story.*

I took my prerequisites. I only had to pass them in order to go to nursing school the next semester. By the middle of the semester, I was "passing" all my courses with a C or better, except for Chemistry. I had a 48/100 at midterm. I kid you not. I think somehow I was actually passing the lab part, but I was nowhere near passing the course.

During the midterm break, I went home. Of course, I had already told my family about how bad my grades were, and I was close to just giving it up. I mean, how would I ever get a 48 back up to a 70? It just didn't compute. My mother, who has always been extremely supportive, didn't tell me I needed to quit—or "you can do this." She didn't placate me and say, "Oh, you don't need to be worried; everything will be fine."

Instead, she spoke symbolically.

When I returned home that night, at the end of our little dirt road leading up to the house, I saw the oak tree covered in yellow ribbons. My mama had gone out and tied yellow ribbons all over it—up on the limbs and around the trunk—for me to see when I came home.

In our family, the song "Tie a Yellow Ribbon Round the Ole Oak Tree"[1] was a big part of our lives. The song's message was basically, "If you still want me, if you still love me after all I have done, just tie a yellow ribbon round the old oak tree. And if it is not there, then I will move on." The storyline says to tie *a single* yellow ribbon, but at the end of the song, there are *many* yellow ribbons.

That is what my mom did. She hung as many ribbons as she could. It was magical to get my first glimpse of all the ribbons and to know instantly that no matter what happened, I could always come home. The choice was mine, to go back or return home, and she was going to love me no matter what. When I saw what she had done for me, I stopped the car and cried. It was an incredible message for a twenty-year-old to be told, symbolically and without discussion—that everything would be okay and I could always come back home.

My mom then told me that if I wanted to quit, I could, but she thought I could do it, so I should go back and at least try. I got all my crying out that week, went back, and gave it my best shot.

Putting everything I had into it, I could only bring my Chemistry grade up to about a 58.

But when the report cards came out four weeks later, there was such a curve in the grading scale that I actually made a C+. Don't ask me to explain how exactly it happened, but it happened. I started nursing school in January 1983 and graduated in December 1984. I took my boards in January 1985 and received a passing score, and my nursing license followed in May 1985. I'd made it.

I can't entirely wrap my head around the FSU/UF thing, or being able to pass all those classes, and certainly not how the curve in my chemistry class could get me a passing grade. But I made it into and through nursing school.

Now here *you* are. Whether you're on the verge of graduating, or have already graduated and are working on your first job, or have been a nurse for years already, it doesn't matter why or how you got here. What matters is that you're here and that you'll help us move nursing forward. And I hope to help you.

CHAPTER THREE

Why Are You a Nurse?

Dear Kasey,

This is a question you'll be asked a million times. And if you're lucky, you already have the answer. I can say that even after all this time, I'm not sure what my answer to this one is. Yes, I've had an answer, but over the years, the answer has changed. But you know what? It doesn't matter. You're a nurse, and you'll make a difference in a lot of people's lives. I can't wait to sit back and watch.

Love, Aunt Kim

What do you want to be when you grow up? No, seriously, what do you want to be?

I know you just graduated from nursing school, but for some of you, that isn't what you originally planned. Hopefully, for some of you, it is.

As I mentioned in the previous chapter, I *never* had any intention of being a nurse when I was growing up. I found out I could go to FSU or UF for a little over two years and get my RN/BSN degree, or I could go back to the LCCC for two years for my RN degree and just get a BSN degree later if needed.

Who knows why I chose the four-year program, but thankfully I did. I've never gone back to further my education. It may be important, and maybe I should have, but I didn't. Yes, I tried to get it started a time or two, but it just wasn't in the cards for me.

I went to nursing school not because it was my dream but because it was job security. No matter what happens in this world, sick people will always need someone to take care of them. It seemed that nursing would be my way of "always having a job." So off I went.

Did I hate it? No. Did it become my passion and fulfill my dreams? Kind of. Did it create job security? Absolutely. It always has and always will. The passion and the love did come—not from the job but from working with patients and their families.

The really cool thing about nursing is that once you finish nursing school and graduate, you can do a million different things. Pass those boards and you can get started in at least a thousand different directions. Think about the jobs in a hospital, and then think about the jobs you can build on to your nursing degree. The computer world is wide open; the business world is wide open; the legal world is wide open. The possibilities are endless.

My career path stayed within the hospital setting, and I held every position from nursing assistant up to nurse manager and/or director. I've been very lucky in my career, and it *was* luck. It had nothing to do with me making great critical decisions at the right time.

When I graduated from nursing school, there were no

job openings in the country for new RNs. My FSU class graduated about sixty nursing students, and none of us had jobs or interviews or opportunities for jobs. You see, in the early 1980s, the federal government and insurance companies developed policies and legislation that would change the future of reimbursement for medical services. The new system was called DRGs, which stood for Disease-Related Groupings. The simple idea was that we would take an average cost for, say, a gallbladder removal, and that's what the hospital would charge and what the insurance companies would pay. The thought behind it was that if you charged a set price (we will go with $5,000 here), it would average out—sometimes the hospital would make money, sometimes they'd break even, and sometimes they'd have to spend a little more than they made. But overall, the idea was that they'd make money.

The hospitals responded by cutting back staff and letting people retire early because the DRGs would change everything. And so they did.

I had worked my way through school, and in my final semester of nursing school, I worked as a student nurse on the Respiratory/Medical floor. My starting salary was $7.35 an hour. The only reason I got a job was that I had worked as an SN (student nurse) and they hired ten of us who had worked through school.

It was actually very cool, one of the first and original nursing internships. We would do a week of study—for example, Neuro-related stuff like ICP (intercranial pressure) monitors, Mannitol doses, head injuries—and then we would spend three weeks in the relevant ICU.

We did this with six units, for six months, and then got

to "pick" a unit. The only shifts available were a few 3 p.m. to 11 p.m. shifts and *lots* of 11 p.m. to 7 a.m. shifts. We didn't have very many twelve-hour shifts available then, and I wish we didn't now.

This all worked out well because it took us three to four months to get our hand-graded board results back. I chose the Neuro unit, and it was one of the best possible decisions with which to begin my nursing career.

Back to the DRGs. Their implementation had led us to release a group of nurses, and because rumor was that nursing jobs would be scarce, the numbers of nursing school applications were reduced for a few semesters—just enough to get us behind.

Since that time in 1985, things have changed so much, and it seems the nursing shortage just continues to get worse. But the fact that people like you are still going to nursing school and coming into the profession to help make a difference is crucial. Thank you so much. The changes you see over the course of your career will be amazing, and who knows—you might find that the reason you're a nurse changes, too.

CHAPTER FOUR

To Help People

Dear Kasey,

I smile when people say, "Oh, you must be such a wonderful, kind, caring person because you're a nurse." I wish that were the truth, but I became a nurse because I knew it was a career where I'd always have a job. As a teenager, somehow I understood the importance of that, and so I went to nursing school. At times in my career, I've been that wonderful, kind, caring person, but that didn't drive my decision. We each have our own reason. It doesn't really matter; what matters is that we are here.

Love, Aunt Kim

When asked why they wanted to become a nurse, most people answer that they want to help people. Okay, that's like Miss America saying she wants world peace.

There are almost as many different reasons as there are nurses. Some hope it'll be exciting work (it often is). Some are attracted to the vast variety of work environments (everything from working at a school to working on a cruise ship). Some like flexible work schedules (night shift, anyone?). Some love the idea of job security (there will always be sick people). Some feel good about working in a well-respected profession (job satisfaction can be a key motivator).

Regardless of the reasons, you found your way to this profession. You're an RN: a Real Nurse. You'll go out and change the world. You'll help cure everyone, watch new life come into this world, and hold the hands of old patients who are gently leaving this world.

Or maybe that's your idealized vision of what you'll do as a nurse. I hate to break it to you, but that's not happening.

I don't mean you won't change the world, but you'll find that what you imagine nursing is like is nowhere close to the reality. And what it means to change the world is a lot less glamorous than perhaps you'd like to believe.

Did they tell you in school that some patients will throw poop at you? That some patients will try to hurt you, maybe even break your arm? Did they tell you that you will end your long, hard shift two hours late and still feel you didn't get everything done?

What if the reality looks more like finally going home and thinking back on this kind of shift: the rude patient in room 16 you couldn't make happy no matter what you did. He was on his call light the entire time. You couldn't do anything right for him or his family. Eventually, when you saw his light on, you had horrible thoughts about how you could "just take care of him like you were supposed to"— and I mean *really* just take care of him.

Then you think on the elderly lady in room 2, for whom you could do absolutely nothing else. She had no family, was alone, and had lived in a nursing home. Instead of making her a "no CRT" (no cardiac resuscitation treatment, which is similar to DNR, or "Do Not Resuscitate") and leaving her at the nursing home to die, they just had to bring her to the hospital. Now she's your problem.

She didn't put on her light but constantly called out for help. She had oxygen on and could barely talk, but she could certainly shout loudly enough. And if someone walked by the door, she'd ask for her sweet little nurse and they'd quickly come to tell you. You quit explaining to everyone why you couldn't keep going in there to see what she needed, because all she needed was for you to sit with her awhile so she wouldn't be alone. If you could just get a few uninterrupted minutes, you could take care of your other patients. The only way the problem—I mean patient—in room 2 would leave was when she died. From the way she kept calling out, it certainly didn't seem like that would happen anytime soon.

You smile when you think of the cute little boy in room 5. He had his Winnie the Pooh pajamas on and was sitting quietly in his daddy's lap because he couldn't move and breathe at the same time. He had his oxygen mask on, not because he was cooperative but because he didn't have the strength to pull it off. He had cystic fibrosis, and there was nothing to do but treat his symptoms. He'd been visiting the hospital more and more because his lungs were getting worse. Each time, you weren't sure if he would make it out. This might very well be his last visit to the hospital.

Maybe the reality of nursing looks like ending your day wondering if there is really a God out there who lets little old ladies live way past their time and be alone in their last days with no one to love them. And who lets six-year-old boys die because they can't breathe. Where are the miracles? Where are the wonderful moments of saving someone's life and knowing you've made a difference?

You can't even think of the last time you had a success story. You've seen too many patients this week with end-stage cancer who want to try just one more time to beat this thing. They want to live, but the cancer has deteriorated their body so badly, you don't even know how they are still alive.

And then it happens. In room 8, there's a thirty-five-year-old mother of two. As you walk in, she's sitting up in bed, her bright pink turban covering what you know is her completely bald head. Her oxygen is on, and she's having difficulty breathing, but modern medicine can do nothing else for her. She's at the end of her short life, and you think about how life isn't fair. Her three-year-old is cuddled up on the bed with her on her left side, and her six-year-old cuddled up on the right—both of them asleep. Her incredibly tired husband sits close by, holding her hand. You walk in to see if she needs anything, and she smiles as she shakes her head and says, "No, I have everything I need right here." You smile back and remind her to call if she needs anything.

You wipe away tears as you shut the door and head to check on another one of your patients. Suddenly, it hits you—you remember exactly why you became a nurse.

In many cases, you can't do anything to improve the lives you touch. Hopefully, you can do something to make them more comfortable, but sometimes there just isn't enough medicine to erase the effects of all the suffering of the world.

Some of your patients will ask for too much; some won't call you when they really should. Some will be sad, some angry. Some will take it out on you, and some will tell you they're fine even when you can see they're crying. Some of them are repeaters who are hooked on drugs or just want attention. Some will live to see another day; some will die on your shift. And some you'll help get better so they can go home.

Some will tell you you're the best nurse on the planet. Others will tell you you're the worst nurse ever. You'll do what you can to help them while you're there. Yes, there might have been better ways to handle that angry patient and family. Yes, you could have tried to sit for longer periods with the dying woman. Yes, you could have done so much more—but you did your best. For most of your patients, you'll never really know if you helped them or not. Yet you'll know you tried, and at the end of your shift, at the end of the day, that's all that matters.

The first few times you were asked why you wanted to be a nurse and you answered, "To help people," you couldn't fully understand what that meant. Only after working some of the worst shifts of your life and seeing some of the worst things in the world, watching people endure things no one should ever have to go through, do you finally understand what "helping people" looks like. And you smile, because that's exactly why you became a nurse.

CHAPTER FIVE

Saving the World

Dear Kasey,

Since I've been writing stories about some of my nursing experiences, my interactions with patients and families, some of my mistakes, and some patient successes, I asked myself why I wanted to write about these experiences. So just as the Grinch sat and thought and thought and thought some more, so did I. Why did I need to recount some of these stories? Do I miss nursing? Do I miss my patients? Do I miss my coworkers? Do I miss being a leader? A resounding yes to all of the above. But the main reason is, I wanted to try to give you an idea of what you were going into. It seems no one can really prepare nursing students for their first experiences as an RN. I wanted to tell you some of my good, bad, and ugly experiences with the hope that maybe, just maybe, they will help you. I hope that in some way they do.

I've watched so many changes in my nursing career, and I know you'll see so much more than I have. The future of health care technology will be amazing. They are making such great strides in so many different areas, and you'll get to be a part of them all. I'm so excited for you.

Love, Aunt Kim

My niece is in her last semester of nursing school. There's so much I want to tell her. The good, the bad, the heartbreaks, the successes—all the ups and downs of my nursing career. There's so much ahead of her, and I can't wait to hear about her experiences. This last year, she texted me when she put in her first NG tube; I let her practice on me for IVs, and she did a great job. I was so proud of her.

Like me, she has a job in a nursing-home-type facility. She's learning so much, and I love hearing her stories about her interactions with patients almost as much as I love remembering my own experiences as a nurse.

One of my favorite stories she's shared is about how she read an article that patients with Parkinson's disease can walk better if they have a song with a steady rhythm. They tried it, and it worked. How exciting! I can't wait to see what additional advances that might lead to in the future.

I've watched so many changes in my nursing career, and I know my niece will see so much more than I. The future of health care technology will be amazing. They are making such great strides in so many different areas, and Kasey will be a part of them all.

I miss nursing. I miss it a lot. The day-to-day smiles of my patients. Seeing someone come into the hospital for a test, worry written all over their faces, and feeling like— by talking to them, listening to them, interacting with them—I can make a difference. Having the repeaters, the ones with long-term illnesses or diseases, say that me being their nurse is making a difference for them. How awesome is that?

Sometimes the difference you make isn't helping them get better; no magic medicine or surgery or test can fix what's wrong. But sometimes I miss just being with them, giving them a hug, holding their hand while they cry—no words needed.

Learning how to do a new procedure, or learning about a new medication. Celebrating with the patient when the test results come back with a good result: that the cancer hasn't spread, or there's no heart disease that requires an operation, or that this time, minimum fluid had to be removed from their abdomen. It all matters.

One patient had terminal cancer and was in the end stages, yet each week his smile was so big and he was so happy. His goal was to set the record for the most amount of fluid ever removed from a patient as his condition continued to deteriorate. The doctors gave him three to six months to live, and he lived well past a year. And yes, he broke the record for the greatest amount of fluid removed from his abdomen—fourteen liters. Think about that. That's seven two-liter bottles of coke. He was so happy about it, and we were happy for him.

Nursing has taught me so much about life—not just how to live but how to die. Watching how people face the end of their lives is amazing. Some fight to the very end, holding on to see a certain family member or for a particular celebration. Some are ready to go whenever it's their time. Some are past ready to go and eagerly await their turn, believing in their hearts that many of their family and friends are waiting for them. They are looking forward to seeing everyone who has been gone for so long—husband, wives, mothers, fathers, sisters, brothers, and pets.

I know I'm talking about my nursing experiences, but you'll learn that once you're a nurse, you're *always* a nurse, even after you leave the hospital, office, or wherever you work. You're constantly reminded of that as family and friends ask you about some "medical" issue and you give them advice, let them know what you think might be going on, explain information they have been told but don't understand.

You'll never not be a nurse. If there's an accident on the road, you'll stop to help. If you're out to dinner and see someone at another table who appears to be in medical distress, you'll go check on them. All sorts of things will come up, and you'll do what needs to be done to help. That's what nursing is all about. That's probably one of the very reasons you chose being a nurse in the first place. And I say again, this crazy, stressful, wonderful career you've chosen will change you in many ways.

There were times I dreaded going to work. It was getting harder and harder to see all the patients around us who were dying and to see family members holding back tears because they had just found out it was cancer or that whatever was wrong wasn't curable. I was frustrated at being unable to help every single person, being unable to fix them all. If I let my mind wander back, face after face comes to mind. There were so many, and realistically, there could be even more.

When I entered nursing school, I thought it was about helping people get better. Now, at the end of my career, that isn't what nursing is about at all. It's about helping people—period. You have to be ready to accept your patient's fate, whatever it is. Sometimes you might not agree with the fate they chose, but you'll be there for them and their family and do what needs to be done. Medicine can't fix them all. You'll lose some, and you'll help save some, but a lot of the faces I flash back to are the ones we lost.

As a new nurse, I wanted to save the world. At the end of my career, I hope when my patients think of me, they think I did my best and that in some small way, I made a difference. I hope when they think of me, maybe, just maybe, they will smile.

CHAPTER SIX

You're Not "Just a Nurse"

Dear Kasey,

I will always support you. I will always try to help you. But I don't ever want to hear you say to me or anyone else, "I'm just a nurse." If you wear a white jacket, all sorts of people will think you're a doctor. I've heard so many nurses answer when asked, "No, I'm just a nurse." There's no such thing as "just a nurse." Nursing is the most amazing career, and nurses have the most amazing talent and knowledge base. We have experiences the doctors will never have because we are at the bedside; we are the ones who call the doctors and tell them when something is wrong. You're not now, and will never be, "just a nurse." If anyone mistakes you for a doctor, just tell them, "No, I'm the nurse."

Love, Aunt Kim

You've been taught again and again about doing an assessment on your patient. You've been taught all the different body systems and sounds to listen to and what questions to ask. But has anyone taught you what to do *anytime* and *every time* you walk into a patient's room? Yeah, we have the usual head-to-toe assessment. But I use something I call the three-minute assessment, which can be done in three minutes or less, every single time you walk into a patient's room—whether it's your patient or not.

It was very important for you to learn how to assess a patient—to learn lung sounds and heart sounds and bowel sounds. You learned it all, and now you have it down pat. You can do a head-to-toe assessment and chart it with the best of them. But after forty years, I've learned a thing or two, and I'd like to teach you one of my little tricks. See what you think.

This is something you can practice all the time—with your patient, with your classmates, at the mall, anytime, anywhere. It doesn't require talking or asking questions; it just requires looking and listening—for anything and everything, honing your skills by being very observant. It's about picking up on both verbal and nonverbal communication. How do people move—do they have a limp, do they walk fast or slow, do they act like they have to concentrate as they are walking? Do they look down, or is their head held high?

The idea is to improve your observation skills so you can use them along with the learned assessment skills you honed during nursing school.

Why? Because as a nurse, you'll walk into a patient's room and have limited time to assess and make a decision about what to do. Sometimes it feels like you only have seconds to make a decision, and in the medical field, seconds *do* matter.

I want to touch on something even more important: the biggest thing you need to learn is how to leave it at the hospital when your shift is over.

If you aren't careful, you'll apply nursing to every aspect of your life. I don't think that's good for any of us, and personally, it hasn't always worked out very well for me.

Don't get me wrong: my three-minute assessment is great for your professional life, and it helps with speedy patient assessments. But using those assessment skills in my personal life wasn't always the best thing. It'll be hard for you to try to separate when you're a nurse from when you aren't—when you need to be and when you don't. Sometimes I rushed into making decisions in my personal life when I should have slowed down and taken time to make a thorough assessment.

Don't get lost in being a nurse. You're so much more than that. Being a nurse is a great thing, but it's not the only thing that makes you who you are. Don't get that confused. You will need to find a way to compartmentalize a bit.

Yes, you'll take patients home with you—no, not literally—but you'll leave the hospital and go home and think about them. And that's okay, but don't let it take over your life. When you're at the hospital, give them everything you can, but when your shift is over, leave it there. There's nothing you can do after you leave. Thinking and planning and wondering and worrying about them won't help them or you. When you go home, leave it there and be fully present at home.

Whether you're by yourself or with your family or friends, that's where you need to be, not back at the hospital. You've chosen this as your career, and believe me, you'll give so much. But an important part of taking care of yourself is leaving work at work. Outside of caring for your patients while you're at the hospital, their struggles are not yours to carry. For some of you, that might come easy, but for others—because of the very things that make you *you*—you'll take it home sometimes, and that won't help anyone.

Go home, leave it, and be "your other self." Be who you need to be to get recharged so that when you go back, you can give it 110%. If you give and give and don't take the time needed for yourself, you'll burn out. You're good at your job, but it's just that—a job. I don't mean to understate the difference you make in the lives of your patients and their families, but to take the best care of them, you must take the best care of you.

Learn this, and learn it fast. You can't give your patients everything, saving nothing for yourself and your family. It's all about balance.

CHAPTER SEVEN

Newbie Nurses

Dear Kasey,

Newbies are my favorite kind of nurses. You've just finished school with all the latest information out in print. You've passed your boards and are excited about this new and wonderful career of nursing. You are our future. It'll be great—a little crazy at times and a little hard, but I think you'll love it.

Love, Aunt Kim

I've worked with nursing students as a preceptor. Their talents and excitement about their career always helped revive my love of nursing.

But to be completely honest, it wasn't until Kasey, my niece (I have two, and I adore them and am so proud of them), decided to go to nursing school that I had the desire to help new nurses. I watched as she worried over care plans and tests and, of course, passing the boards. My own daughter, Megan, chose to be a pediatric occupational therapist, and I'm so happy for her, but she's in uncharted waters for me. But I watch her developing and advancing within her career, and I think it's so amazing when people find their niche. Believe me, Megan has found hers.

Bailey (my other niece) came out of school and went straight to work. She is in a customer service business and seems to be promoted daily! She has moved about five hours from home and is very happy and successful. All the "girls" are doing great.

But let's get back to Kasey going to nursing school. I was terrified because I knew what this child was going through. I knew what it felt like to be genuinely afraid that I hadn't passed boards. I knew that being exposed to the world of nursing would put her in situations it's difficult to prepare for. I wanted to help her and other newbie nurses by telling them some of my experiences and hoping it would in some way help them deal with the amazing things that lie in front of them and their careers.

Let's be honest, going through nursing school is a bitch. Sorry, but there really is no other word to describe clinicals, tests, classes, and boards. But when you get through school, *don't panic* about boards. You've been storing all that information in your brain, and even though you might not think so, it's there. Go take those boards with confidence. You're finished with school, and for a lot of you, this is the start of your lifelong dream career. For others, you'll finally be making good money. Don't worry, don't stress, and remember—*it doesn't matter what your score is.* It's a pass or fail. As long as you get the magic number right, you're in with the rest of us.

Clinicals can be a wild ride. Many nursing schools start everyone out in their first clinical at a nursing home. Looking back on it, I love that we get to start there. We are all so excited about the opportunity to begin caring for patients, and although nursing homes are, unfortunately, one of the more underserved areas, the patient you've been assigned often gets one-on-one attention all day. When you're choosing where you want to work, look for teaching hospitals. They are willing to let people learn and make mistakes, as long as the patient isn't placed in any danger. Many people working there are happy to have the help and to play a role in the future of health care. One of these new people—whether new RN graduates, residents, or new doctors—might just hold the magic key for some of our biggest discoveries in health care. It's an amazing opportunity.

During the interview, you're not the only one being interviewed. They are interviewing you to see if you're a good fit for them, but you must also interview them to decide whether they're a good fit for you. The nurse manager interviewing you deserves your respect. Sure, they have been there, working and taking care of patients, but you went through school just like them. You passed the same tests, boards, and clinicals, so you also deserve their respect for what you've been through.

Your nurse manager will play an important role in your life. She will be the one you go to for time off; when you've had an incident; when you have a family crisis and need time off; when you need support, motivation, and someone who will listen.

I also like when my nurse manager knows almost as much about the care of the patients in her unit as her staff does. That way, if you run into an issue, she can be right there in the thick of things and be part of the solution. I never wanted someone criticizing me for my work if they had no idea what I was doing, much less were able to do the job themselves. However, I was blessed with all my nurse managers, and I hope I made a difference in the world of my staff.

If the nurse manager isn't in the room, ask what it's like working for that person. Ask what working with the team is like. Ask what the turnover rate is. Ask anything you like, because this will be *your* team. This isn't about money, the "place to be" in the hospital, or "the team to be on." This is about finding your place in this world, where you can be the most valuable asset possible. It takes many of us several times to get it right. Some of us get out of nursing school and know exactly what type of nursing we're interested in. We just have to figure out which hospital or unit.

I had no idea and bounced around various jobs and roles. That's the great thing about nursing—if you don't know, try it. You may be like Little Mikey and like it (though you might be too young for that reference).

I can honestly say that if they had offered to double my salary to take a position in the Labor and Delivery unit, I'd have turned it down because that wasn't the right fit for me. Folks, if you've tried it and discovered you don't like it, more money won't make you like it. You might go to work, and you might get through the day, but if the passion isn't there, you're wasting your time.

Find your place. I believe most people ask you to stay at least six months, maybe one year, when you commit to a position. But if it's not a good fit for you, try another unit. Do you realize how many different units exist? Then take into account the different shifts and the possibilities seem endless. It's exciting!

A big part of your new job is to lean on your fellow staff members. Ask questions, and *observe* what they do and how they care for their patients. You may find that your team members do things differently. We all develop a unique way of doing things. There's nothing wrong with that as long as when the patient is transferred, sent to surgery, or discharged, everything that needs to be done has been done.

Every unit has a variety of staff: women, men, young new nurses, older new nurses, and all different ages of experienced nurses. They all come from different places and backgrounds and are from all over the world. Everyone brings something unique with them to the team. The long-term, experienced ones have not only seen a lot of changes but have also been through rough times as nurses.

The numbers say there's a nursing shortage, but I don't agree. Due to all the changes in health care, we have had to pull a lot of RNs away from taking care of patients to the business side of the career for charting, documentation, and payment. The good news for you is that it leaves a lot of bedside positions open. The bad news for health care is it takes nurses away from direct patient care.

We are way better at nurse-to-patient ratio than we use to be. When I was young, I heard older people say, "You have it so lucky—you don't know what tough is. When I was growing up, I had to walk uphill both ways to get to school." I'd roll my eyes. I thought it was funny then, and I still think it's funny now.

Likewise, in nursing, all of us "old-timers" will say you

have it easy. Or at least, we used to think that. You new-bies know more about the computer and charting than we do. That's why it's so cool to put a newbie, who can spin around the computer with ease, with an oldie who can spin around a patient and in seconds realize what they need. It's great to combine the old and the new.

Now that I'm the "old" one, I understand they were try-ing to tell us (in their own unique way) things had changed a lot. Progress had been made, and we had it much easier than they did. I completely agree with them.

There used to be a saying: "Nurses eat their young" (more on that in the next chapter). I know it's true because I've talked to *many* nursing students who feel the staff nurses don't want them there. We are overwhelmed. It's not you, so don't take it personally, but we have all of our usual work to do, *plus* (and this is a *huge* plus) we have to put all the information into the computer and then help teach the newbies. We often feel overwhelmed by every-thing that needs to be done. But the last people this should be taken out on are the new nurses coming in to help us.

By the way, please take the nickname *newbie* as a com-pliment. I'm very excited about all the new nurses coming out of school, familiar with computers and having all sorts of new and exciting ideas about nursing care. I can't wait to see what all of you will do with that fresh energy and your innovative ideas.

You're entering nursing at a time when a lot of great job opportunities exist, the technology is changing fast, and the skill set of the nurse is advancing with the tech-nology. In five years, so many things will be better for patients and for the nursing staff. It's hard for those of us not familiar with the technology world, but all of you grew up with it. We need each other.

I'm as excited for you beginning your career as I am about my retirement. Hang on to your stethoscopes—it'll be a wild and exciting ride!

CHAPTER EIGHT

Nurses Eat Their Young

Dear Kasey,

I wish it weren't true. But unfortunately, it is. For the life of me, I can't understand why when we are so short-staffed and need help, experienced older working nurses will treat the newbie nurses as if they don't know anything. Well, of course they don't—they just got out of nursing school, and they need us experienced nurses to help them learn the ropes. Please try to understand that in general, nurses are overworked and feel they don't have enough time to take care of their patients, much less a newbie who has questions. But don't let that discourage you. There are great preceptors out there, and we're glad you're here. But it's one more thing on our plate. The culture is changing. Hang in there. We will all get through this together.

Love, Aunt Kim

It's true. We nurses have been working our butts off for years, and I'm here to tell you we don't have time. You've heard about it—you know there's a nursing short-age. You know a lot of nurses have been overworked for years and the last dang thing they want is a greenhorn they have to teach how to blow their own nose. Many working nurses just don't have time. I mean, you've seen what they have to do. You get to take your care plan home and research and think about it. Meanwhile, the nurse you just left on shift must finish all her documentation today, and that includes a care plan including all the stuff you just looked up.

We know a lot, and we know a lot of shortcuts, but we don't know it all. You need to learn all we know—I liked when newbies asked questions. But I liked it better if they thought about it and tried to figure it out. It would also be better for them to make a note to ask me at a different time, rather than when I'm up to my eyeballs taking care of a patient.

One of the biggest crises right now is how extremely overworked nurses are. They don't want to take time to help the new kids on the block learn everything. Older nurses should be supportive of the younger nurses, but what can the younger nurses do? The older nurses want respect and appreciation for their experience. It's not that they want it to be stated, but they want it to be shown. Therefore, new nurses offering to help is a big deal, even though the experienced nurse may not need it at the moment.

My advice to young nurses is, even if you have a break, offer to help if you see everyone is busy. Most of the time, they will say no, but the fact that you offered makes a world of difference, because they feel you are paying attention and that gives them encouragement. It makes all the difference in the world because you are not sitting down when no one else has a chance to sit down. That would make it look like you are not a team player or you are not willing to work. I understand that you're tired and need it, but everybody else does, too. So ask.

Also, when you are on the floor, the experienced nurses don't want to cram a lesson down your throat. They want to know that you know what is happening. So when someone says they're going to do a procedure, you as a newbie say, "Hey, can I go watch and help you"? Volunteering to do that matters, whether they tell you yes or no, because they see you're trying to get more knowledge and experience. It makes a big difference to the experienced nurses that you are actively trying to participate instead of leaving them to ask if anyone wants to get some new experience.

I absolutely want you to know everything I know. Do you know why? Because one day, I won't be able to do this, and I want to make dang sure you're a *better* nurse than me when you take care of my family—or, at some point, me. I want you to know it all, but sometimes I just don't have the strength or patience or time to tell you, especially in the hectic moment you're trying to ask me. I want you to know, and I want to teach you, but *help* me teach you.

CHAPTER NINE

Paving the Way to the Future

Dear Kasey,

Over your career, you'll meet nurses from all walks of life, with many different experiences, and even from different countries. Each one of them will in some way teach you something. And all of us, regardless of how long we have been a nurse or what type of nursing we have done, have something to offer. Try to remember that, because the older experienced nurses may sound rough at times. It's because they have been through a lot and seen a lot. The newer nurses have the advantage of new stuff that they just learned in school. And everyone in between has had experiences. Everyone has something to teach you, and all you have to do is pay attention. Maybe you won't like what you learn from them, but it'll still be important information.

Love, Aunt Kim

Throughout my nursing career, there have been good and bad experiences. Now, at the end of my career, I can honestly say it's the good ones I remember most. I've been able to draw on so many different memories to help newbie nurses with difficult or challenging issues. While some have been what many people may consider bad or hard or negative, I don't agree, because life is about living and learning. Whatever you learn helps you with the next patient or helps you grow as an individual. Therefore, I don't think we should refer to any experience as bad.

Throughout my career, I ran into many opportunities and made more than my fair share of poor decisions. However, I was very lucky because when I made those decisions, I had great mentors, role models, and most importantly, great supervisors who helped me through them.

You know, it's true what they say: whatever rough time you're going through right now is only preparing you and propelling you to the next amazing adventure. But at the time, it certainly doesn't seem that way. In the middle of surviving, all you can think about is surviving. I certainly never thought, *"Oh, no bother, things will be amazing after I get through this bullshit."*

But life is about making mistakes. If you aren't making mistakes, it's often observed, you aren't learning or growing. I believe that's true for most people, though some people are born with the gift of avoiding mistakes. I personally know several people who are that way, and they completely baffle me.

In the movie *WarGames*, a powerful new computer is able to make the decision of whether to fire the first missile from the United States to set off a nuclear war. Matthew Broderick's character hacks into this government computer and accidentally initiates a nuclear war scenario. But when the kid asks the computer to play tic-tac-toe against itself, it realizes that both tic-tac-toe and nuclear war result in no-win outcomes, so it shuts down the missile launch.[2]

The reason I bring up the movie is that most of us are like that computer: we just have to try something for ourselves to "see what happens." I'm one of those people, and I don't regret it. You have to jump out there and try something, anything, even if it's wrong. Maybe do what someone else tells you is absolutely wrong, just to make sure. *So what* if they are wrong? What if this time, when you try it, it works and is absolutely the best thing in the world? What if it completely changes direct patient care?

Thomas Edison emphasized that he had learned several thousand ways *not* to make a light bulb.[3] But the whole time, he was actually working toward the magic combination that would allow him to perfect it. Think about that for a minute.

Yeah, I'm old, and I know that "things have changed." I can tell you a million things we do now within nursing that we would never have considered doing before. But in making those changes, we've improved the care of our patients. We've included the families (fathers weren't allowed in the room for the birth of their children); we've improved our patient outcomes (e.g., we now tightly control everyone's blood sugar during surgery, whether they are a diabetic or not); we've made the patient and family the center of the experience (which seems sort of obvious now); and we've made a health care team rather than a "know it all" doctor-oriented plan of care. Each of us has a role to play in the care of the patients, and yes, that includes the patient, their family, doctors, nurses, techs, pharmacists, dietary, environmental care, maintenance, and everyone else it takes to "keep the lights on."

What you do as a nurse today has the power to make a difference. You never know what will come from the work you do. Perhaps even your mistakes are paving the way to a better future.

CHAPTER TEN

A Change of Scenery

Dear Kasey,

When I retired for that short year, you know that I got into Uber and Lyft driving. I loved it. A lot of people think it's because my passengers were trapped in the car with me and I could talk, and they had no choice but to listen unless they wanted to jump out of a moving car. It was similar to nursing in that I met all sorts of people—some nice, some not so nice—and the experience gave me a new perspective on things. You never know in life what will happen and how things will change you. But I promise, it's always interesting.

Love, Aunt Kim

About a year ago, I retired from nursing. I wasn't really burnt out or tired of it, but I had the opportunity to retire, so I did. Okay, thinking back, maybe I was a little burnt out. The Kim in my head started talking way too much, and I was afraid she'd end up saying some things out loud that are best kept in my "inside voice," as I like to call it.

I realized I had been doing some form of nursing for forty years, so it was a nice round number. Maybe I wanted to step back and review my life. Maybe it was a midlife crisis. Who knows, but I found myself moving from Tallahassee to the Orlando area and, of all things, I started ride-sharing—as in, driving people places. I needed to get out of the house because the person I lived with worked from home, and I was not very good at keeping busy or quiet. I safely delivered people from point A to point B for four months, and I *loved it*.

I often told my riders I had retired from nursing and switched to ride-sharing because I'm very quiet and shy. But it doesn't take anyone very long to figure out that obviously, I'm not quiet or shy. *Quiet* is a word that has never been used to describe me in any situation.

One day, I had a series of stops and starts in getting my first riders, but the drop-off zone left me in downtown Orlando in the area I will now forever refer to as the Convention Corner. It seems that maybe every other driver in the area knew it but me. That day, however, would seem to be a bit of irony for my future because a week-long convention was going on called National Teaching Institute 2019 Critical Care Nurse Exposition.

I picked up numerous nurses/riders there from all over the country, and even though most of the trips lasted less than fifteen minutes, I talked to them. No matter the years of experience or where they were from, all of us agreed there's a crisis within nursing and that we needed to keep our newbie nurses happy so they would stay with us in our units.

The interesting thing was that some of them were surprised to hear how high the national average turnover is and some of them weren't surprised at all. We discussed why we thought it was an issue. These conversations gave me additional insights about why newbie nurses don't always stay the full first year in their new job.

The most important thing I learned was that the shortage was happening all over the country. I spoke to nurses from as far away as California, South Dakota, and Illinois. It was amazing to talk to all these nurses and hear the *exact* same thing. And the one thing that scared me most was that *none* of the twenty-plus nurses said that money was the issue. The same thing over and over was that newbie nurses want a very different career path than what we had.

New nurses are desperately needed in nursing—not just a warm body but *you*. Each nurse brings so many things to the table when they are a bedside nurse. The patients need that. And we as the aging population of nurses need that. We need to see the excitement and enthusiasm and the new, fresh ideas you bring to the table.

But most importantly we—veteran nurses—need you—newbie nurses—to try to understand where we have come from and what we have been through and understand that we are excited you're working with us. But sometimes, we are just over it. We say things and do things and make facial expressions that should have stayed with our "inside voices." We are tired. We are worried and hurting and frustrated. We want to do as much as we did before and work however much we need to work to help cover, but we really are tired. We know you're here to help us. We are worried that we will spend all this time training you and you'll just leave because we know there's always another job. But we want you to stay here with us.

In my opinion, there's really no lack of RNs, just a lack of RNs at the bedside. Due to "paperwork" and "billing" and "insurance," a lot of great RNs are actually somewhere pouring over paperwork so we can get reimbursed. You hear that a hospital has X number of nurses, but guess what? With management positions, teaching positions, insurance verification, chart review, IT positions, and countless other positions, fewer nurses are at the bedside to do direct patient care. Advanced technology requires RNs to be in the room for procedures like they already are for surgery.

I usually tell anyone interested in nursing, "There are so many opportunities within the nursing field." Now that I'm back at the bedside, doing direct patient care, I've changed my battle charge to, "That's great, we need more people like you at the bedside to help care for patients."

Now, before I get into trouble with all those who are doing important jobs away from direct patient care, I want to say this: We have got to, as a profession, "figure this out." We have to work together so we can be motivating to you newbies and get you to come into the profession not just because we desperately need you but because we, as a profession, love it and want others to be called to do the job with us.

But over and over, I hear newbie nurses say they want to leave because they can't stand the way they are treated in their unit. And it's from their coworkers right on up through management.

One reason I went into nursing was because I knew I'd always have a job opportunity. I knew that while it might not be excellent pay, it would be good pay. But make no mistake, it's hard. Your patients are sick. The hours are rough, and we always need extra help, or extra hours, or extra anything.

And just like with the nurses I met while ride-sharing, no one yet has said that the single thing that will make a difference is more money. Yes, we all could use it and it certainly won't hurt, but it doesn't seem to be the solution.

We need you to talk to us; we need your voices to be heard; we need to know your thoughts and ideas of how to change nursing so that it's a career we can all enjoy and work together to make it an amazing, fun—yes, I said *fun*—job. You should enjoy your career and be excited about it and the opportunities you have in it. I know we deal with sick people, but it's a career nonetheless, and we need to be excited about it.

So what do you say? Will you help us do that? Will you be the change and help that we need to propel this career into the future and make it a dream career with all the trimmings?

I know you can.

CHAPTER ELEVEN

Infusaports

Dear Kasey,

I smile when I think of you starting those IVs on me. It was so cool to watch you trying and learning and listening to my advice. I was so excited when you got a blood return. I actually think I was more excited than you because I realized what a big deal it is. You'll have to learn procedures, and so many new things on the horizon will be different and will challenge you. But I'm not worried a bit. You'll be great at learning all of it.

Love, Aunt Kim

With all of these advancements happening in the world of medicine—the very ones you are going to be a part of ushering in—it can sometimes be daunting for us seasoned nurses. It's not always easing to adapt to the constantly changing landscape. Let me give you an example.

"Hey, Kim, can you take the patient in room 401? I just arrived on the nursing unit to start my shift. I don't drink coffee, so I can't say that I'm fully awake, but I'm here.

She will be quick and easy; all she's here for is a 2000cc infusion of Ringers Lactate," said the charge nurse, handing me a chart.

Sounded simple enough.

"Sure," I answered the charge nurse. So I grabbed the chart and headed to the med room to get my supplies. Down to the room I went and knocked as I entered the room, saying hello to my "quick and easy" patient.

As I entered, I was doing my quick "once over" assessment as we talked. She was a very pleasant lady in her mid-fifties; seemed to be in good health. No problems breathing, alert and oriented. I asked her if she was ready to get started and she nodded.

As I sat next to her with my supplies, she said, "Oh, didn't they tell you, I have a port."

I tried not to let any emotions show, but I noticed my hand had stopped in midair, halfway to the patient's arm. I was speechless and terrified. "*Oh no*," I thought, "*not a port.*" I could feel myself starting to sweat; I told myself to take slow, easy breaths.

I managed a weak smile and said, "That's great. Let me go get a few more supplies and I'll be right back."

I quickly left the room, leaning against the wall as I tried to get air back into my lungs. Now with the way I was acting, you would think the patient had just told me she had a highly contagious disease with no cure or treatment and less than three months to live, and I've just been exposed. Okay, okay, I'm being dramatic, but I have to be completely honest and tell you that my *biggest* fear is that I'll do something to kill someone. I've never even come close, but it just seemed that somehow, someway, I would screw up beyond all belief and do something with horrible outcomes.

Remember in nursing school, you got to see all sorts of amazing technology and advances in medicine. True, the bedpan and the patient gown hasn't changed at all in the last one-hundred years, but everything else is changing rapidly, and as a nurse, you struggle to learn how to use, insert, read, control, turn on, turn off, access, de-access, and countless other techniques to use the "new equipment," use needles, give the medications, and keep up with all the techniques, making sure you are doing everything exactly right, *every* time.

Computers came along and made our lives easier, but we didn't stay caught up so that all our technology could talk to one another and we could see what everyone else was doing with the same patient. Part of the patient's chart is in one system, part is in another system, and yet part of it is still in a hard copy chart. Yes, that's right, real paper that has to have those damn holes punched in them. Then the fun really begins when you drop the chart and half of it spills out on the floor; part of the hole is ripped; and it needs to be thinned because you can't find anything in it. Someone wants to know where the EKG result is from four months ago. Heck, I can't even find the paper copy of the one done this morning.

I've seen so many machines hooked up to a patient that you could barely see the patient at all. It looked like the bed was full of wires and tubes and lines. You could hardly get to where the patient's head was because of all the machines around them. Then you, as the nurse, need to know not only how to work every machine but you also have to know about all the different meds you're giving.

So many advances have made a difference for our patients, and for me, infusaports are one of them. The use of infusaports has given us an amazing way to access an IV line for our patients unlike the old way of having to stick them until we get good IV access. I can remember, as an ICU nurse, sticking patients and sticking them and sticking them some more. When they are very sick and have been in the hospital for a while, you have to find a good IV site. My own mom was once stuck thirteen times just for a simple fifteen-minute outpatient eye surgery. Getting the IV took longer than the procedure!

Then came the invention of infusaports. They're small devices implanted surgically (by the surgeon, not us—thank goodness) that then can be used to draw blood or give fluids. They're usually used for chemotherapy.

Do you ever feel like you went from nursing school and learned about all these amazing things and then get out in the real world and realize, *"Oh, crap; they expect me to do it."* I was always trained and had a preceptor, but it always freaked me out when it was my turn to actually put in a Foley catheter, NG tube, or IV. And now we have added these wonderful, overwhelming new access lines; like central lines, and PICC lines, and, of course, the infusaport.

I can honestly say that accessing them *now* is no big deal, but the first three to four times, I was very nervous. No, nervous isn't the correct word—terrified. You gather all your supplies and go into the room and explain what you'll be doing and then, it's time. You have to actually access the line.

Now, let's think about the fact that the patient has probably had this done, numerous times. I bet they could even access their own lines, and most of them know what should and shouldn't be done. I think that's very important, but it doesn't help my nerves any knowing that the patient knows more about what I'm about to do than I do.

This has happened to me throughout my entire career. It's not that I'm insecure or don't think I can do it; it's just terrifying that I'm doing something that, if not done correctly, could possibly kill a patient. They could get an infection if I don't use an absolutely correct sterile procedure. If everything isn't flushed and primed correctly, they could get an air embolism that could kill them. Yeah, a lot of things run through our minds that could go wrong, but throughout my forty years, none of them has ever happened.

Earlier I talked about inserting IVs. To me, that's a piece of cake compared to the completely sterile technique of accessing an infusaport.

I can name at least twenty things I can do wrong just while setting up for the procedure. First, you make sure to open the sterile package correctly to avoid touching or contaminating it. Next comes opening all the sterile packages that are needed but not part of the original sterile package. Then you have to empty them on the sterile field. Somehow, it seems something always hits against the sterile field and rolls off. You know what that means. Grab another one. Hopefully, you have an extra, if not, you have to leave the room. But before you can do that, you have to close up the sterile field to make sure it doesn't get contaminated. Next are the sterile gloves. I'd love to have a contest where everyone puts on their sterile gloves. Come on—how hard can it be? But it is.

Next comes setting everything up on the tray. Don't reach too far or your sleeve might extend over the sterile field. It's difficult opening some things because of the sterile glove, but you can only open things on the sterile field with sterile gloves on. Are you kidding me? It's complicated just writing about it!

I smile when I think of my first few times. But you'll get better and you won't do anything that someone else hasn't done before you. I mean, how hard is it to open a 10cc syringe and drop it in the middle of the sterile field? Pretty easy, right? Unless it hits the needle package and then ever so slowly rolls to the edge of the field and right off the edge of the table and onto the floor.

And all of this is being done in front of a patient who, again, probably knows more about how to do it than you do, and you're the trained nurse.

Remember that all of us have to learn how to do something for the first time and have to practice to get really good at it. And these days, new devices and procedures are coming up all the time, so it's a constant learning curve. Just remember that all of us had to learn it and are still learning it. Do the best you can, and keep trying. That nurse with twenty years of experience is learning some of this at the same time you are.

Oh yeah, and as for accessing that first port? I aced it, and I'm now the Queen of Infusaports.

CHAPTER TWELVE

Nurse Take Two

Dear Kasey,

In writing this book for you, I've realized something. Since I went back to work after retiring for almost a year and since you just graduated and are just starting out on your career, we are kinda in the same boat. We are both in our own way newbie nurses. Kinda funny when you think about it. Kinda cool too.

Love, Aunt Kim

I've retired two or three times now.

I had been a nurse for over twenty-eight years when I retired the first time. The first five of those years was as a bedside, neuro ICU nurse. I loved it and learned a lot. ICU bedside nursing is what I "cut my teeth" on. But the years led me in a managing direction and away from the bedside. Yes, it was important to me to be able to care for the same patients as my staff did, and I kept my hands-on care approach as much as possible. I pulled night call in the PACU to keep my skills up to date and acceptable. But I didn't do it every day like the staff did, and there was a difference.

I didn't know just how much of a difference until I decided, after twenty-eight years, to go back to my roots. I went back to the beginning, back to bedside nursing. Boy was I in for a surprise. I was about to feel like a newbie all over again. So when I say I understand what you're going through, I mean it.

I took a position back on the OPSU where I had been a nurse manager at one time. This had been one of my choices in my first ten years of nursing, so I thought I'd be a little rusty. But I also thought it would be just like riding a bike; it would all come back to me.

What I didn't think through was the fact that everything had changed. We were now doing our charting online; meds were dispensed through the electronic pyxis machine; neither the Foley catheter kit nor the IV start kit was anywhere near the same. Okay, the IV start kit did have a needle in it, but that was about the only thing similar. In fact, thinking back, there was no IV start kit, we just grabbed the appropriate-sized needle, a tourniquet, and some wipes and got started. Nothing like the nice, neat, all-in-one little packages we have now. What a great improvement these IV start kits are.

However, when you take this great kit to the bedside, it does nothing to improve your aim or skill at hitting, threading, and securing those evasive little veins. It's nothing like riding a bike. Going back to the bedside after being away from it for over twenty years is like going from crawling directly to riding a bike. You'll have to learn, relearn, or practice a whole bunch of stuff in between. It doesn't just come right back.

I didn't realize I was a newbie nurse all over again until about a week into my orientation. I found myself with some of the very same feelings I had as a new nurse, fresh out of college. I felt like I knew nothing.

I had been a nurse manager for most of my career, had been able to care for patients at the bedside in a limited capacity, and was a "leader" for my staff, but that doesn't add up to a lot when you're told that the patient in room 1 needs an eighteen-gauge needle with fluids started in both arms. Eighteen-gauge? Two of them? Both arms? I felt like I had just been told to paint a masterpiece in three minutes. What I was being asked to do was *impossible*. Wasn't someone going to show me, wasn't someone going to let me watch at least ten being performed before they turned me loose on a real patient? What was going on here? Didn't they know I might injure this patient if they turned me loose by myself?

The preceptor asked if I thought I could handle it. I don't know how long I stood there and looked at her; I'm guessing my mouth was still open from when it dropped open immediately after I realized what she had just asked me to do. She continued, "You're an experienced nurse, right?"

When no sound came out of my open mouth, she handed me my cute little compact, complete IV starter kit, and the necessary eighteen-gauge needles and pointed toward the room. As I turned to walk in that direction, I could barely hear her as she said, "Just let me know if you need any help."

That was the longest walk of my life, and it was only two doors down.

I walked into the room, washed my hands, introduced myself, and checked the armband. I told the patient I needed to start an IV on her as well as draw some blood to get her ready for surgery.

I felt like I was in a daze, but I grabbed a chair, sat down by her bed, and opened the new little kit. I thought to myself as I laid out the supplies, *"Well, would you look at that. Everything I need is right here in this little kit."* I placed the tourniquet on her right arm and, as silently as possible, took in a deep breath.

Right there in the subcubital area was a huge vein. I could see it immediately. I put on my gloves, glanced at the makeshift table I had set up on the patient to make sure I had everything I needed, and warned her that she would feel a stick.

I pushed the needle in, and blood returned; I released the needle and threaded the little catheter in. I wanted to jump for joy, but I still had to draw the needed blood vials and get it taped down, which took a few minutes, and then I was through. After I finished tapping it, I so wanted to throw my hands up like I had just scored a touchdown. I wanted to do a dance in the end zone for my success. But all I could do was smile inside, look at the patient, and say, "Okay, that wasn't so bad. Let's get that other one started."

We have so many procedures to do during our career. Some, like IVs, we become such pros at it that we could literally do them with our eyes closed. But many procedures are more complex, and we do them so infrequently that it makes us feel like newbies each time we do it. When you feel that way, know that it's in your head. You know what you're doing. You've been taught how to do it, and you may have even done it a few times. For any procedure, make sure you have at least had it explained to you, get your supplies, hold your head up high, walk into that room, and do your thing.

CHAPTER THIRTEEN

Be a Team Player

Dear Kasey,

So many people assume so many things. You've heard about the legislator who said nurses just sit around and play cards. A lot of people will walk up and see a situation and make an assumption. Don't be one of those people. We don't like it when patients and families assume things about our days, and it's just as important, or maybe more important, for us not to assume it about our team members.

Always try to give people the benefit of the doubt. It will serve you well, because in so many situations, we really don't know the whole story.

Love Aunt Kim

Like in the military, your nursing team is called a unit. That "fighting" unit can run if all the people are there. Things happen and parts of the units shift and change, but the core is there: the belief in each other, in doing what's right, in doing whatever needs to be done to get the job done.

As a manager, I once walked up to the unit and heard a

patient on the call light asking if someone could take them to the bathroom. The person who answered said that, yes, she'd send someone right down. There were several nurses at the desk who didn't budge. I paused for a few minutes, acting like I was looking at today's paper. I waited about a minute and then asked, "What room was that patient in who needed to go to the bathroom?" I was told, and I went down to the room.

On my way down, two of the people at the desk told me they'd take care of it. I told them not to bother, that I had it. I assisted the person to the bathroom, and then I went back to the desk. I'm pretty sure the message was received because no one was at the desk whose job didn't require them to be there.

Now let's talk about that for a minute. I walked up to the desk and I had no idea what the last hour had been like. This might have been the first few minutes the team had to catch their breath. It was, after all, only like a minute. I didn't look at each person to see what they were or weren't doing. I admit that I was mad at first, but I had no right to be because I couldn't make a judgment on what was going on by standing there for only one minute.

However, I could make a judgment that I, as the nurse manager, had the time to stop and take that patient to the bathroom. We won't go into salaries here because there's no need to. How much it "cost the hospital" for a nurse manager to take a patient to the bathroom is irrelevant. The hospital would pay me the same amount to sit there and glance at today's paper as they did for me to help a patient to the bathroom. I needed to give my staff the benefit of the doubt because that's what a team does. I assume they have a reason and it's a really good one. They don't need to take the time to explain it to me, nor do I need to waste time with them telling me. They are my team and that should be good enough.

As a newbie nurse, you will learn the flow of the unit. You will learn that it has been slow for the last hour and then for the next two hours, it will be hectic. It may be one of those days when no one gets to have a break or lunch. Don't make yourself the exception. Make yourself the person that sets the example by offering to help everybody.

CHAPTER FOURTEEN

Everyone Is on the Same Team

Dear Kasey,

You'll do a million different things to make a difference in the lives of the patients and the people on your broader team you come in contact with. But nothing, absolutely nothing, will make a difference more than the simplest thing in the world—a smile. You have a beautiful smile, and as a nurse, you need to show it, even if sometimes on the inside you don't feel it. I promise you that it'll make a difference.

Love, Aunt Kim

Back in 1911 in New York City, the people who pick up trash decided to go on strike. What does that have to do with nursing? *Everything.* They didn't feel their work was being valued, they didn't think they got enough pay, and they wanted additional benefits. So they went on strike in one of the biggest cities in America for nine days.

Everyone in the hospital is there for the patients. Even if they never see a single patient, they are in the hospital to help it run smoothly. For just a moment, think about how many people in your department aren't doing nursing jobs—unit secretaries, environmental services, someone in room 5 fixing a light, another person in green working on the water in the main patient bathroom. If you pay attention to just one shift (even a night shift), you'll realize it takes an army to take care of our patients.

The nurses get the attention. Sometimes, it's not even the type of attention they want but when you think of patients, the first place anyone's mind goes to is nursing. But what about environmental services, food services, pharmacy, therapy, transporters, and all so many others. Every hospital has numerous departments. Where's all this help? Behind the scenes making sure that you can do your job. If any of those departments shut down for just a shift, it would affect your ability to take care of "our" patients.

We all need to recognize that it takes this army to care for our patients. Without this support system, our jobs would be so much harder and, in some cases, impossible. I'll review just a few examples.

Unit secretaries. They know what's going on with all the patients on your floor. You want to know where a patient is? Don't check with the charge nurse; check with the unit secretary. They know what's happening and truly have their finger on the unit's pulse. Anytime they "tell you something," pay attention—they're telling you for a reason, and it's not just to "bother" you.

Nurse techs. They go by a lot of names, but again, they are very important to you. They probably see your patients more than you do, and if they tell you something is going on with the patient in room 12, you need to go see. They know.

Environmental services (ES). Without them, the

hospital would look similar to New York City in the strike of 1911.

Not only are the people on your unit valuable to the care of the patient, but so are the people all over the hospital on other units, in unseen offices and areas you might not even know about.

And here's the thing. You get the highest salary. You get paid the best. Nurses get the raises. Nurses get the attention. But you couldn't do a thing without everyone who is working with you and working behind the scenes so that we can care for our patients.

When on your next shift, notice who is there with you. Think about who they are, why they are there, and how they might affect your ability to do your job. I know that sometimes we think, or unfortunately say, something like, "Well, if Pharmacy would just send up my medicine faster, I could take better care of my patients." That's true, but Pharmacy has to send up everyone's medications. You have six patients. They have to cover the entire hospital, including the Emergency Department.

I hear things like, "Environmental Services (ES) did a lousy job cleaning this floor," and I cringe. Not because it's not true, because it is. But what do you know about the people in ES and what they have to do? I don't like cleaning my own house, much less having a job where I'm cleaning up someone else's "house"—cleaning up behind them, washing their laundry, mopping their floors, emptying their garbage. Do you enjoy cooking or having to "serve" someone, clear their table, and wash their dishes? That's not a job for me, but *someone* is doing it. In fact, it takes a lot of someones to get the job done.

Now there's something very important I want you to do. I can hear you saying now, *"Oh, good lord, now what is she wanting me to do?"* It's very simple and quick, and it won't hurt you at all. *Smile* at everyone. Say hello to them as you walk by. Thank them. Help them in little ways to show that you notice what they're doing.

It seems like every single time I want to go grab a sip of my Coke from the break room, ES has just mopped it. Some people just walk right on in and make tracks all through the hard work they have just done. When I was a little girl, I got a spanking if I walked on my hardworking mother's freshly mopped floor. Honestly, I never did it because nothing made my mama madder than for someone to walk across a floor she had just worked very hard to clean. How often do you mop your own house? ES mops our break room every day.

The other day, I was heading into the break room and the woman had just finished mopping the floor. She said, "It's okay; you can get what you need." I told her that as a little girl, I'd have gotten a spanking and that I wasn't about to walk on her clean, wet floor. Then I paused and said, "Thank you so much for mopping it for us every day."

Her smile lit up the room and for the rest of the day, every time I saw her, she'd smile at me. And since that day, when I see her, she smiles and asks if I've gotten a spanking yet.

When our CEO walks down the hallway, you may see him stop and pick something up off the floor. He does it all the time. Since becoming the CEO, he has taught us that keeping the hospital clean is everyone's job and that

ES needs all of our help. So take a minute to pick things up off the floor in the hallways. When caring for your patients, put the trash in the trash. Help out in the little ways and it'll be noticed. I'm not asking you to do their jobs. I'm asking you to do yours. As a child, we are taught to clean up after ourselves—putting our trash in the trash, not leaving things lying around. It's so important in a hospital to help each other out with the basic things.

But if nothing else, when maintenance comes in to change the light, thank them. If it has taken three weeks for them to get to it, don't make any snide comments. Someone is here now. Smile and thank them.

I've often heard that it takes more muscles to frown than it does to smile. Whether that's true or not is irrelevant. What's important is that when you smile at someone, you're acknowledging that you see them, that they are noticed, and that you're happy they are there.

Your support system and people on your team are not there to help you. They are doing a very important job in helping to take care of the patients. Their jobs are just as important as yours. Yeah, I heard that: *"No way; you're crazy; they can't do what I do."* And yes, all of that's true. But you couldn't do what you do if they didn't do what they do.

CHAPTER FIFTEEN

Down and Out

Dear Kasey,

One of the most amazing things about nursing is that so many different opportunities exist, and anyone can find a place they love within the nursing field. I love hearing when nursing students know exactly where they want to work. Some of us don't find our niche until later. But it seems at some point we all find it. Here's to you finding yours sooner than later.

Love, Aunt Kim

For those of you who hit nursing school knowing you want to be a Labor and Delivery nurse or even a newborn or pediatric nurse, my prayers have been answered. I've never been able to deal with either one of those areas. Having never had a baby, I don't understand what the patient is going through, and I just can't bring myself to start an IV on a child. The other day one of my coworkers said she was really good at putting IVs in babies' heads—they call them scalp IVs. I about threw up just hearing about it.

While in nursing school, my Labor and Delivery

experience and my Pediatric Psych experience both about
did me in. For example, I was assigned to a laboring patient for about six hours. The husband and family were
very supportive, and I was told by my nursing instructor
that I had gotten a "good one" because she wasn't screaming and yelling the entire time. I don't know about *not*
screaming and yelling, because the thought of giving birth
to an eight-pound bouncing baby did seem to me that
screaming and yelling would be involved.

I provided what "support" I could by refreshing the
cool, wet washcloth she kept on her head, by helping her
in and out of the bed because she never could seem to get
comfortable, and by taking her back and forth to the bathroom, which seemed to be a constant thing. As a young
nurse, each time I took her to the bathroom, all the "stories" I had read about babies being born and falling into
the toilet came rushing back to me. But I'm thankful to
this day that the baby didn't fall into the toilet.

I was watching the labor wave form on the monitor, the
baby's heart rate, and the mother and her coach as they
breathed through another labor pain when my nursing instructor slipped into the room. She motioned me over and
whispered in my ear, "Your shift is over." For a simple
two seconds, I was so excited—until she continued, "But
she's so close to birth, I've made arrangements for us to
stay." I knew she was expecting sheer excitement at this
wonderful opportunity that so many of my classmates
would have loved to have. I mustered up a quick thanks
and turned slowly back to my laboring family.

The labor and delivery nurse came back in, I tried to
stay up by the patient's head when the nurse announced,

"Let's check things out and see how we are doing."

"*Yeah, let's do that*," I thought. Then she motioned for me to come down to where she was. I quickly changed my mind about "checking it out."

After only a few seconds, the nurse quickly jumped up, pulled off her gloves, and ran to the phone, paging overhead, "Any doctor to labor and delivery room 5, *stat!*" Then she quickly turned back to the patient and family and said, "We are about to have this baby."

I felt like I had just started the downhill ride on the world's largest roller coaster. My stomach was going crazy, and I promised myself I *wouldn't throw up* at the sight of a baby being born. As a farm girl, I can't tell you how many puppies, kittens, cows, goats, pigs, and horses I've watched being born. But this was a *baby*. I felt my stomach lurch again as if we were taking a fast turn on that roller coaster ride.

I watched in amazement as nurses came in and efficiently set the room up, positioned the patient, and got the warming lights for the baby all the while talking very calmly to the patient and family. I was not only way out of my comfort zone, but my expertise had long ago been passed by. I was standing in a corner trying to stay out of the way and wishing with all my might that the coke and crackers I had eaten earlier would stay where they were. But it was questionable at this point.

In just a few minutes, the doctor came in, all gowned and gloved, and announced, "Let's get that baby out of there." Everyone took their positions, and even though I was comfortable in my own little corner (like Cinderella), my instructor insisted on me standing behind the doctor so I could see everything. I was nodding my head yes, I could see just find from where I was, as she pulled me by the arm to position me behind the doctor, and it took everything I had not to run from the room.

I noticed when the instructor had positioned me to where she thought I could best see, she sort of pushed down on my shoulders. I assumed she was on to me and was trying to secure me in place as best she could. She, however, got to back up against the wall, in my spot.

Now things started to happen, and I actually began to feel myself becoming excited. While I was pretty sure this wouldn't be my future path for nursing, I was about to see a baby being born.

That time is forever etched in my memory. The baby's head was crowning. Everyone in the room was excited, and I joined in. I would be one of the first people *in the world* to ever see this little baby. It was so exciting, and I could hardly wait.

The doctor said, "If you can just give me one more big push, I will perform the little cut procedure like we talked about and this little one will be here."

What? I had read about this in the books, but no one had spoken to me about it. It's called an *episiotomy*, where the doctor does a cut on the mom's perineum so there's a decreased chance of the mom tearing as the baby is being born. Very clean and simple is what the textbook said.

Things happened so quickly that all I can tell you about the next ten minutes is that the very soon-to-be mom sat up, grabbed her knees, and looked like she was about to push an elephant out. As the mom pushed, the head of the baby slowly eased out and the doctor very gently took the scissors and made a simple cut on the mom, just above where the baby's head was coming out.

Okay, that's it—that's all I have for you.

"Wait, wait, wait," you say, "what happened, was it a boy or girl, how much did it weigh, how did the mom do?"

Sorry, folks, but I can't help you. You see, that was the first, but not the last, time I found out that in this wonderful new career I had chosen, the one thing that would make me lose it, the one thing that would time and time again be my undoing, was "nice, clean incisions." Yup, I can handle everything else—trauma patients, open fractures, extensive wounds, infected wounds, and anything else that has crossed my path in the last forty years, but I can't watch a clean incision and not pass out.

Now a clean incision to me is an incision or cut with a knife type instrument along a nice smooth piece of skin. No blood is involved (well I can't say that really because I've never seen what happens immediately after the cut). It's a controlled, expected, usually planned event, but my brain can't handle it.

I passed out during the episiotomy, while watching a nice planned carotid endarterectomy surgery, and also while I was a part of the sterile field for an incision on a lower leg to relieve the pressure from compartment syndrome.

I've been told that one minute I'm fine and the next minute I'm slowly sliding to the floor. Apparently, the instructor laughed at me, the physician who had asked me to watch his surgery yelled for someone to catch me (I was on a step stool, again positioned so I'd have the best view), and the neurosurgeon I was assisting with the compartment syndrome issue merely asked someone to hold the leg and protect the sterile field since "she's apparently passing out."

I know nurses who are terrified of needles, faint at the sight of blood, and politely vomit as they hold the container for their patient to throw up in. Every nurse I know has something. Apparently, I was blessed with two because besides fainting at the sight of nice incisions, I also have issues with respiratory secretions (snot)—but that's for another day.

I wasn't part of the magic of this baby's birth. I wasn't one of the first people in the world to ever see its little face. When I got up off the floor, the baby was laying wrapped in its mother's arms. Life was the way it should be.

What do I want you to learn from this story?

We all have our weaknesses and limits. One day in your future (if nursing school didn't teach you what it was), you'll find it.

Not all nurses will admit to a "career-related weakness." That's okay, but just remember they have it, and one day if you work together long enough, you'll learn about it or maybe even be witness to it. Try not to laugh and try very hard to be supportive. Some of us have some pretty weird ones, but it is what it is.

One of the hardest lessons you will learn as a nurse is the patient always comes first, even if you are uncomfortable, if you are hurt, if you have a stomachache, if your toe hurts—no matter what you feel.

Learn to appreciate the humor. That makes it a whole lot more fun.

Remember, we all have our embarrassing weaknesses. No matter what yours happens to be, you will still be a successful nurse.

CHAPTER SIXTEEN

Smiling Sammy

Dear Kasey,

So many patients will come into your world, and you'll re-member a lot of them for a lot of different reasons. But as you go through this wonderful new world, try to look for the positive and happy times, with whoever you're working with. This patient could have been someone I felt sorry for, but I smile every time I think of him. May you have many memories of patients who make you smile.

Love, Aunt Kim

On my first day with Sammy, I received a change of shift report. I was updated on his vitals, medications, and the fact that his injury was a gunshot wound to the head and the shooter had still not been apprehended. I was told he was awake and pleasant, and the nurse smiled and said, "He's also a character." I was to find out that simple de-scription was a *huge* understatement.

Sometimes when patients come into the hospital from an accident, we don't have the opportunity to "get to know" them—who they are and what they're like. That's why families are so important because as we are caring for an unconscious patient, we get to know the family and through them, the patient.

When he had first come into the hospital, he was unconscious, rushed to surgery, and it had taken a few days for him to wake up. For my shift, he was awake and seemed alert and ready to go.

And then the reports said he'd have severe brain damage and when he woke up, he might have limited movement or thinking abilities. Wrong again. He woke up completely normal—moving all extremities, oriented to person and place, but a little fuzzy on time. He had complete memory recall except for a short time right before the shooting. He could remember only some of the days in the hospital, but other than that, his memory was intact. This was all great news, but we would soon learn he didn't quite get everything back.

After the report, I reviewed the meds and saw that none were due at this time. I went to his room and introduced myself to the officer assigned. Because of the memory loss at the time of the shooting, he had no idea who'd shot him, so he had an officer stationed outside his door in case the shooter wanted to come back and finish the job.

Sitting up in bed, he looked like anything except a patient. He was awake, alert, and when I introduced myself to him, he smiled the biggest smile ever, told me his name was Sammy, and said, "Nice to meet you."

I told him I would be his nurse for the day and would do his assessment. With a brain injury patient, you always start with their neuro assessment to see if there's a change in the status. Being unable to remember things he had remembered the previous shift could indicate a problem. So I began the assessment, as always, by asking his name, date of birth, the current year, and where he was. He answered every question appropriately. Then I explained I'd be listening to his heart and lungs next. He said, "Certainly."

I put my stethoscope in my ears, leaned over the rail, and placed the end on his chest. I asked him to breathe deeply as I listened over each area of the lung, and he did as I asked. Next, I told him I would listen to his heart and he could just breathe normal. As I listened to the familiar and steady heart rate, the patient slowly reached up with both hands and very carefully grabbed my boobs. No, I don't have big overwhelming tatas—but they are a grabable size.

I stood up and looked at him, and I'll admit, I was taken aback and maybe even a little perturbed. But he was my patient, and this had to be handled professionally. Patients are not allowed to grab nurses' boobs—no exceptions. I asked if he understood that what he had just done was not appropriate and not allowed.

As I stood beside his bed, looking down at him, waiting for his answer and certainly an apology, I was surprised by the look on his face. This man was in his fifties or sixties, but he had the facial expression of a four- or five-year-old boy. Then he replied, "But they are so nice and soft."

I was thrown completely off guard. His responses didn't make it seem sexual or aggressive. He sounded like he was only explaining why he had done something. It seemed he didn't truly understand that he'd done anything wrong. He lowered his head and in the slightest of voices said, "I'm sorry; I won't do it again."

This was my first interaction with a grown man whose injury had changed him forever—but in a way that would only show itself at certain times. Upon meeting him, you may never know he had an injury unless the opportunity presented itself. The residual effect of his injury was that he had no inhibitions. *None.* If he wanted to pick his nose in front of you, he did, not to make you uncomfortable but just because he felt like his nose needed picking. Somehow the injury had taken away the part of his thinking that allowed him to know what was appropriate or inappropriate, what to do or not do, or what to say or not say based on the situation.

In forty years, this is the only time I've seen this type of result with an injury. I've heard of similar stories, but this was my one and only firsthand experience with it.

This was a huge challenge for his family because they were embarrassed by his actions, which is totally understandable. This was a grown man who they felt "knew better," but that part of the man was gone forever.

It was hard to watch as the family tried to deal with it and the patient get upset that he'd said or done something to upset his family or any of us. He wasn't trying to; he just didn't have any inhibitions.

For the rest of his stay with us, I always asked to have him as my patient. I understood him, and even though he was inappropriate at times, he was very sweet. And he always wore that great big smile.

I often thought of him in my head as Thumper, the little rabbit in *Bambi* who got caught eating the "flowers and not the leaves" of the blossoms. When Thumper's mom asked him, "Thumper, what did your father tell you?"[4] Thumper always answered her with an innocent voice. The innocent voice of Thumper is the same voice I'd hear from my patient when he'd say, "I'm sorry. I know I'm not supposed to...." Then he'd tell me bluntly which unacceptable behavior he had committed. It was horrible, sad, and cute all at the same time.

I could have been strict with this man for his inappropriateness, but I could tell he didn't mean to misbehave. It was like the little boy in him had come back and there was no way for him, or any of us, to help the little boy learn how to grow back up.

He evidently went home with his family fully functional in every way. I've often wondered what their life was like. The family so embarrassed by the actions of a grown man (as I'm sure most of us would be). And the grown man so sad about doing something that made his family unhappy or disappointed.

Eventually, they found out it was a family member who had shot him. The patient thankfully never remembered that, and I think it's a good thing. But the entire family had to pay for the actions of one member, and their lives were changed forever.

My experience interacting with this patient was embarrassing at times, but he could always make me smile because he wasn't being mean or sexual. He was just being himself—without a filter and without the brain function that allowed him to process what was socially appropriate.

He was one of the happiest people I've ever met. His

world was forever changed, but thankfully a beautiful part of him remained—that wonderful, beautiful smile I got to see every time I went into his room. His cheerful disposition despite everything he'd gone through.

You'll see so many things throughout your career. Be careful to not be too judgmental. You never know the whole story.

You'll have so many adventures in this great nursing career you've chosen, and each one will teach you something.

CHAPTER SEVENTEEN

Oops

Dear Kasey,

I love you and think you're amazing, but you're not perfect. None of us are. We all make mistakes as nurses. It's okay because you're human and no one is perfect. All you can offer your patients is to do the best you can do.

Love, Aunt Kim

Let's talk about my first drug error.

I can just hear you thinking, *"Oh no, did the patient die? Were you fired? What did it do to the patient? Was your license suspended?"*

Hold on, hold on—I will tell you.

Regarding your future in nursing, I'm not so sure your life will be easier than mine. We did the best we could with what we had, but we didn't have computers to chart on, dispense medication, or record the armband and drug information on the patient.

We were left to our own methods of double-checking and being very careful, and yet, sometimes it still happened. We would make a drug error. As scary as it sounds, it's the truth.

I was working in ICU at the time, and we had an orange cart that had probably twenty to thirty drawers on it. We had ten beds/patients in the ICU, and each room/patient had a drawer with their name and room number on it. Now the drawers didn't lock at all. When you checked the Medication Administration Record (MAR) and saw what medications were due, you opened the correct labeled drawer, grabbed the medication (back then we knew a lot of medications not just by their label but by the color of the pop-off tab), poured the ordered amount in the medication cup (this was a liquid medication), and went to the room and gave it to the patient.

Let's talk about patient assignment here, just so you have a little bit more information.

When I worked in the ICU, there were two RNs, two LPNs, and ten patients. I had just passed my boards and was a brand new "baby nurse," as new nurses are sometimes referred to. And I was working the dreaded night shift—7 p.m. to 7 a.m. I was solely responsible for my two patients and also assigned to give the meds to the LPN's three assigned patients. So that gave me a total of five patients whose medications I was responsible for.

Most patients' meds are via IV since the patients are usually critical and unconscious. But all patients in the ICU are in different levels of recovery, so some of them weren't as sick as others and were waking up, getting better, and would soon be discharged from the ICU to the floor.

That explains how I had a patient with a PO (by mouth)

liquid medication. One patient had mostly IV medications and a few PO meds. However, he was unconscious and couldn't swallow, so I'd be giving it through the NG tube, which is that awful tube they put down your nose into your stomach. The other patient had a few IV medications and some PO medications. The LPN's patients had a few IV meds, however most of theirs were PO, which the LPNs would give at the scheduled time.

Medications were assigned at regular intervals to help us keep up with the time. To this day, I don't believe a better system has been developed. Medications which were needed every 6 hours were given at 6 a.m., 12 p.m., 6 p.m., and 12 midnight. Medications given two times a day (b.i.d. meds) were given at 6 a.m. and 6 p.m. The first dose for medications would be due at 6 a.m., regardless of how often they were scheduled. So every two hours, we needed to check the MAR to see if any of our patients had meds due.

As stated, I was responsible for five patients' medications as well as hourly vital signs and assessments, turning and positioning, and bathing. It never made sense to me to bathe a confused patient in the middle of the night. It doesn't seem conducive to helping them get oriented to time. I mean, who takes a bath at 2 or 3 a.m.? But that was the deal.

On this particular evening—the evening on which said medication error occurred—it was midnight and all five patients had scheduled medications. So I pulled open the first drawer and saw that only one PO medication was due. I put it in the mediation cup and walked to the appropriate patient's room. Or so I thought.

When I got to the patient's bedside, I proceeded with his PO. I saw that he had an NG tube in place, so I checked to make sure it was positioned correctly. You do this by listening to the stomach with your stethoscope while pushing a 50cc syringe full of air into the air vent located on the side of the tube. If it's in the proper place, you'll hear it bubble. With the tube placement verified, I poured the med down the NG tube, flushed it with a little water, replaced the stopper, and left the room. I don't remember whether the patient was awake or alert or if I talked to him as I gave him the medication. I guess the shock of finding out later what I had done would erase all of those memories from my mind.

I won't go into all the reasons why this happened, could happen, or why it shouldn't have happened, but the bottom line is that it did. Let's just say that we didn't check and double-check armbands then like we do now. And we certainly didn't have computers to double-check for us.

So I went back to the "med cart" to pull up the next patient's meds and realized my mistake. I had just given bed 2's PO medications to the patient in bed 3. Uh oh. *I absolutely, beyond a shadow of a doubt, knew I'd just killed the patient in bed 3.* He would be having a cardiac and respiratory arrest any minute now. I was surprised that I hadn't already heard the monitors going off, signaling to the entire unit my horrible mistake.

I *ran* back into the room and looked at my patient. Absolutely nothing had changed. He was exactly as he had been since I came on shift at 7 p.m. Vitals stable, breathing on his own, and from the looks of him, resting quietly.

How could this be though?

Without wasting any more precious time—time necessary to save the patient instead of trying to figure out why he wasn't dead yet—I rushed out to tell the other RN, the "charge" nurse, fearing the worst. She'd have to call the head nurse in the middle of the night and tell her what I had done, and she'd come in and fire me—not to mention the fact that the doctor would be called to rush in and pump the patient's stomach to remove the medication and save the patient from the very jaws of death.

As the charge nurse listened to my report of having given bed 2's Tagamet to the patient in bed 3, I braced for the obvious horrible reaction that was to come.

She looked up from bathing her patient and said, "Just go get some more Tagamet, give it to the patient in bed 2, and write up an incident report." I was so stunned that I just stood there with my mouth open—not fully comprehending what she was saying. Why weren't we on the phone calling everyone? Where was the team that would save my patient from me killing him or, at the very least, making him sicker?

The charge nurse looked back up at me and asked, "Is there anything else?" I slowly let my breath out, shook my head no, and went back to the med cart. I don't remember much about the rest of that shift except checking and rechecking and rechecking each and every medication. I was so vigilant about it that I can't even tell you how many times I checked each medication that night. Let's just say, I believe that was the longest night of my life.

The next morning, after giving a report and "confessing" to the day shift how I gave the patient the wrong medication and he had miraculously survived, I shuffled to the head nurse's door to receive my punishment. I made sure I'd done absolutely everything so after she fired me, I could just run out the door, clock out, and head home to figure out how in the world I could ever support myself now.

The only thing the head nurse said was, "Did you write up an incident report?" I nodded but still couldn't bring myself to look her in the face.

And then she said words I can still hear in my head, words that have stayed with me throughout my forty years of nursing: "Did the patient die?"

For a minute, I couldn't answer, but finally, I shook my head.

She then said, "Learn from your mistakes and move on. We all make mistakes; we are human. We have chosen a career where we have the opportunity to make a difference in people's lives by helping them. But at times, we may make a mistake. All we can do is try to keep from making the same mistake again. Now go home and get some sleep and we will see you tonight." That was it. That was everything said about my medication error. I couldn't believe it.

Learn from my mistake, and make sure you do everything you can to always do the right thing in every moment you are on the job as a nurse. But remember we are all human—and humans sometimes make mistakes. We now have protocol in place: we utilize scanners to scan the patients' bracelets and scan the medication, and then the computer confirms it is the right medication at the right time for the right patient. If you are following these steps and honoring the protocol—the very protocol put in place to save you from making the same mistake I made—it is nearly impossible to make a medication error. When you do your job to follow these processes, it protects the patient *and you.*

When nurses make mistakes, and they will make mistakes, it is helpful for them to distinguish whether it was the process, or whether it was the nurse's mistake. While there's protocol in place to keep you from making mistakes, I also acknowledge that sometimes circumstances in the nursing world force you to do things that aren't always the right thing. Sometimes there's an emergency and the seconds it would take to scan the patient's bracelet may be the seconds that decide between life and death. And sometimes in those emergency moments, mistakes are made.

Sometimes those mistakes are harmless, sometimes they are mildly harmful, and sometimes they kill a patient. That's the reality of this environment where oftentimes life is hanging in the balance.

I promise you that when you make a mistake, you will never forget that day. And more than likely, you will never make that mistake again. Take that mistake and learn from it, not just in that circumstance, but in a wide-variety of medical events.

It sucks to make mistakes. But you can't go back; you can't undo that error. All you can do is learn from it and move on.

CHAPTER EIGHTEEN

I Got It

Dear Kasey,

Welcome to the world of nursing. You made it through nursing school, and now on to the real world. You'll see it all. You'll see so many more advances in technology both for the patient and for you as the nurse. I hope that with this story, you'll see that the most unexpected things will happen. Some will make you laugh, and some will make you cry. And this particular story always brings a smile to my face. I can't wait to hear your stories.

Love, Aunt Kim

I should have begun this book with a fabulous story about some dramatic thing I did that changed a patient's life forever. Something so incredible that just by itself, it'll leave you begging for more. Perhaps a patient interaction that shows caring and compassion? Or an amazing story with a little drama thrown in for good measure—you know, suspense. Something that leaves you asking, *"Will the patient make it? Will the nurse save the patient from the brink of death?"*

Let me just write about the first patient I remember caring for. I want to highlight the minimum possible number of patients I've seen in my career. Say I averaged working twenty-five hours a week and there are fifty-two weeks in a year, and let's say I saw on average five patients a day (in my dreams). That makes a grand total of twenty-five patients a week over the course of forty years.

That's at least 52,000 patients that I took care of, spoke to, or helped—or who possibly yelled at me or had some other type of nursing-appropriate interaction with me. A lot of patients, a lot of years, a lot of interactions, yet I've never forgotten who I consider my first patient.

He was an older man who needed medication on his uncircumcised penis. I was a nurse's aide at the time, and the nurse on duty told me to go in and "help the patient" put the salve on his penis. She handed me a small tube and said, "Let me know if you need any help" as she turned back to her medication cart. She had given me my assignment and now expected me to complete it.

I turned around and walked very confidently toward the patient's room, knowing I could help this man put some salve on his penis. It sounded simple enough. Keep in mind that I grew up on a farm surrounded by lots and lots of animals, so I had seen a few things in my life.

I walked into the patient's room where he was sitting completely dressed in a chair by his bed. I introduced myself and told him it was time for his salve (as I held up the tube in my hand) and that I was here to help him. He said, "Thank you for coming to help" and quickly stood up and started unbuckling his pants.

Maybe the thought has already occurred to you, but at

the time, I didn't do much thinking before walking down to his room to "complete my assigned duty." But let's think about this for a minute. I'm going into the room to help this man put salve on something that's basically sitting in his lap. He can get up and get dressed, and now that I've seen him, he can stand and apparently ambulate all by himself. Right—after forty years, I can see a little bit of an issue here, but I had walked into that room with confidence and hadn't thought about it that much. I knew that I could handle it; I was a tough farm girl.

As he pulled his pants and underwear down around his knees, he slowly turned and sat on the edge of the bed, looked up at me and said, "Are you ready?"

To which I quickly replied, "Yes, sir."

I looked at his groin area and realized there was nothing in sight. Yes, you heard me. I see nothing. No penis, no nothing. He ever so slowly reached down with both hands and pushed on what appeared to be his pelvic area. I was watching the entire time, and for just a fraction of a second, I saw something small and flesh-colored pop up from the bottom of his abdomen and then disappear just as quickly as it appeared.

The patient looked up at me and said, "You missed it."

I don't know if I stood there by the bed for a few seconds, minutes, or hours. I do know that I had been prepared for a lot of things, but not for what I saw. I'd say it was about the size of your pointer finger. It had popped up and then disappeared before I could blink.

The patient said, "Let's try this again. When I push down, you grab it and hold it until I can get a hold of it, okay?"

I quickly replied, "Yes, sir."

I had helped my dad work cattle on our farm and had been run over, kicked, pushed, stepped on, and knocked down by thousand-pound animals. I was tough, and I wasn't about to let something *little* like this get past me again. I knew that this time when it popped up, I'd grab it and hold on for dear life, just as I did when those cows tried to get past me.

He looked up at me and again said, "Ready?"

I nodded, thinking, *"I've never been more ready in my life."*

It all happened so fast, but this time when he pushed down and the little thing "popped" up again, I reached down, quick as lightning, and grabbed the end of it, holding on for dear life. The patient said in an excited voice, "Hold on to it until I grab it below your fingers."

I will tell you I had no intention of letting this thing get away from me again; I held on tight.

The patient held it with the thumb and pointer finger of both hands on each side and looked up at me, smiled, and said, "Now we got it."

While he held it, I unscrewed the top and squirted some of the salve on the end of it, and he pulled his fingers away and said, "There we go now," as again it completely disappeared.

I remember this patient clear as a bell, and I will never forget him. But I was given a job and I accomplished my nursing assignment, assisting my patient with putting salve on his penis.

What lessons do you think this one experience taught me? Surely you can come up with a few.

You really never know what you're walking into when you're meeting and interacting with a patient for the first time, so be ready for anything. Master your control over your composer, facial expressions, and emotional reactions. Even in the most unusual situations, you don't want to make your patient feel uncomfortable—even if you feel unbelievably uncomfortable.

New nurses have a lot to learn. Don't place pressure on yourself when you meet a new challenge with a patient. You aren't supposed to know everything; you're supposed to learn new things all the time. And your nursing career will teach you that and a lot more.

Whatever you decide is the best approach, do it. You'll either learn what works or what doesn't.

CHAPTER NINETEEN

All Patients Matter

Dear Kasey,

Life isn't fair. Life is good, and exciting and amazing and sad and a lot of other things, but it isn't fair. When life isn't fair, if you can, do something to change it. If you can't, learn how to cope with it and don't let it burn you out or make you bitter. There will be good days and bad days, and good people and bad people. That's life. But they all matter, and in your career, you'll learn that the hard way and probably be more aware of it in nursing than in any other career you could have chosen. But with the good and the bad, it'll be an amazing trip.

Love, Aunt Kim

Over the years, we in the medical profession have very much become a true team with all of us working together for the patients. Nurses, doctors, therapists, techs, and all the other people needed to make it work. My advice is to never ever forget they are there. They are the reason that the whole thing runs and works. Without them, the people working directly with the patients couldn't do their jobs. Never underestimate anyone working within the hospital setting; they are your lifeline enabling you to do what you do.

We are dealing with people at some of their lowest, saddest, most difficult times in their lives. Their emotions run every way possible—laughing, crying, screaming, yelling, running away. Patients and their families are doing what they can, in the best way they can deal with whatever is going on in their life. And we have to stand there and take it and help them. A line is drawn that patients and their families can't cross, but you as a nurse get to decide what you can and can't tolerate. But please keep in mind that no matter what, they are in a hospital setting and that's a place no one wants to end up.

I was working as a floor nurse giving IV infusions when I met Mr. V. He said he was Iranian and had been in the country for two years. This patient had a horribly debilitating disease and needed an infusion to be able to function.

I got him checked in and ordered his medication from the pharmacy. I informed him it had to be mixed in the pharmacy and would be sent up as soon as it was ready. It should have taken about forty-five minutes, but three hours later, it still wasn't there.

While I was in another patient's room, Mr. V. went up to the desk to ask if we could find out what was going on and how much longer it would be. Needless to say, he was very upset about the delay. But the nurse he was talking to felt like his anger was misdirected and that he was being pushy. He was standing at the desk (she was sitting down) and she said she felt threatened.

She called a code grey, which is what we do if we are

dealing with a violent or potentially violent person. I heard the code overhead and came out of my patient's room and saw Mr. V at the desk. He was angry and waving his arms and talking loudly. I completely understand why the nurse called the code. But this was my patient, and I knew the circumstances behind his frustration.

I gently touched his arm and asked him to please come back to the room with me and we would get it fixed. He followed me down the hall, and we entered his room just as I saw five security men and an administrator coming down the hall. I was very thankful that he didn't see them. I gently told him I would step just outside the door to handle getting his meds and I'd be back in less than a minute to finish talking to him.

I stepped out into the hall and explained to the security team that I had things under control. To give you some perspective of the social and political climate at the time, it was right after 9/11, at the height of the Osama Bin Laden issue. They said they weren't leaving until they knew everything was fine, and I asked them to wait at the nurses' desk and assured them that I'd pull the emergency light if I was uncomfortable.

As I entered the room and went to close the door behind me, Mr. V saw all the officers and became very upset. He said we had called security on him because he was from Iran, that we were mistreating him and delaying his treatment because he was not an American.

He was yelling but not threatening in any way. I told him it was okay to feel whatever he was feeling, but it wasn't okay to yell. He needed to calm down so we could talk and that he and I would get this fixed. He paced around the room. I told him I wasn't afraid of him, no matter where he was from, and that I understood why he was so upset. I asked what I could do to help him calm down so we could talk and figure out the best solution.

It was then that he told me why he was so upset. You see, because of current circumstances in the world, his little boy had some issues with some kids at school. And if he had to wait after school for any length of time, he got picked on and, in some cases, pushed around. He had told his son that he'd be there today when the bell rang so he didn't have to wait. And now because of the delay in getting the infusion, he would be late. He wouldn't be there for his little boy, to protect him and take care of him. Yes, he was angry. Yes, he was frustrated—but now do you understand why? There was more to the story than him simply being frustrated by a delay.

While we were in the room talking, his meds came and I was able to get them infused, and he left in time to pick up his son. But so many different things were going on that none of us really saw the whole picture.

Pharmacy had a misunderstanding as to who was mixing the medicine. I wasn't following up every thirty minutes like I should have to help fix the problem because I was busy with a chemo patient who was nauseated and throwing up. The charge nurse was doing the best she could, but she probably shouldn't have even been at work that day because her son was in the military and there had been a huge incident overseas and she hadn't heard from him. And the patient was worried about his little boy.

As a nurse, it can be like that every day. I remember the incident vividly, perhaps especially because at the time I'm writing this, it's the eighteenth anniversary of the 9/11 attack.

As a nurse when you walk into a room, you probably know the patient's name and diagnosis but nothing else. If it's a car crash, you don't know if someone was killed in the wreck with them; if they were beaten, you don't know the circumstances behind the attack. I can give you thousands of stories where what I (or we) thought was going on really wasn't the situation. But as humans, we do make certain assumptions.

When you walk into the room, you're there to care for whatever might be wrong with that patient. Try to focus on just the patient and the job in front of you. Leave the other thoughts and feelings at the door. You just never really know what the whole story is, and the rest shouldn't matter to you. But you're human, and if after caring for the patient, you have to take a minute and go somewhere and cry, or be angry or sad, do it. But don't walk into that room as anything but a nurse there to do everything you can for that person. That's your job. They are your patient, and that's all that matters in that moment and time.

We are all human, all of us, and the most vulnerable person in the circle is the patient. We say the patient is always right, and that's true. But I'd like to amend that to say: the patient is always right; *however*, their perception of what's going on may not be right.

It's late at night and the patient is trying to sleep. All they can hear is the laughing at the desk. They think not only is the nursing staff just goofing off, but they are being so noisy they're keeping their patients from getting valuable sleep. They need that sleep because only a few minutes after the patient falls asleep, the nurse will come in and ask them if they need a sleeping pill. The patient thinks, "*No, if you had just quit laughing earlier, I'd have already been sleeping.*"

But what's on the other side of the door? What's really going on at the nurse's station? Do you know? Do you want to know? Do you even care? Or is all that matters that you didn't get to sleep?

It matters what's on both sides of the door. At least that's what I think. Any unit at the hospital has a lot of sadness but also a lot of hope and good things happening. However, people are usually not in the hospital for a good reason.

We help people get better, or at least well enough to go home or go to another facility, and sometimes we help them face the reality of dying.

Those nurses you hear laughing should try to be a little quieter so the patients can get some rest. But they just finished a code down the hall, and they lost a patient. They aren't laughing because they don't care, or saying, "Oh, well, there went another one." They need to laugh about something positive and funny to get through the rest of the shift without absolutely losing it over the fact that they just lost the twenty-six-year-old father of two to cancer after caring for him for over six months. Maybe they'd grown to know him, care for him, and yes, even love him. They watched when his kids came into the room and he struggled for the strength to smile and play with them as they climbed on his bed, not letting them see that he had just rated his pain a seven on the pain scale even after all the pain meds we had given him.

Maybe they are laughing about a funny story that the patient who just died had told, reliving it together in memory of him to keep a part of him still with them.

Nurses often laugh to keep from crying. With all the things we see every single day, it's amazing to me that we all keep coming back and keep trying to make a difference in the lives of patients and families. When they win, we win; when they lose, we lose.

But when a patient dies, the family goes home to deal with it the best they can, and the nurses just go into the next room, hoping we made a difference for that patient and family while they were here. And as we push open the door to the next patient's room, we are thinking maybe, just maybe, this time we will help the patient and family win whatever battle they are fighting. *Maybe*—because there's always another patient and always another battle.

CHAPTER TWENTY

Fresh Water

Dear Kasey,

As a nurse, not just a new nurse, some days you'll feel like you just can't get everything done. But all you can do is be your best. Remember that the patients are doing the best that they can in their situation, even though sometimes we may think, "Why don't they just deal with it; it's not that bad." I can't say there will be more good days than bad days, but remember, all you can do each shift is the best that you can.

Love, Aunt Kim

I was sitting in a restaurant and overheard someone telling their friends that once when they were in the hospital, they waited an hour to get some water after they had surgery. I know if someone has had nothing by mouth (NPO, *nil per os*) since before surgery, getting some nice, cool water sounds better than anything in the world. But I don't think the nurse was sitting at the desk catching up on the hospital gossip. I think she could have been in a thousand different places, trying to take care of her patients.

I once couldn't give a patient water like she asked. Was it because I didn't care? No. You see, I also had a patient who'd had a diagnostic lung test that day, and he was having trouble breathing and wasn't looking good. I also had a chemotherapy patient who, despite all the medications we gave her, couldn't get rid of her nausea. I also had a patient at the end of the hall, who had been screaming for the past three hours, scared of the people in the room who she thought would get her, although she was the only one who could see them.

As a nurse with three to five patients, you have to prioritize, and it's not that you don't want to bring water to the post-op patient. It's that you have to prioritize—breathing first, nausea second, confusion third, and then the water.

But by the time I get everyone settled down, it's time to check on the post-op patient's pain med and see if it helped any. When I stop by to check on him, he doesn't look good and says something doesn't feel right. And let me just add here, if a patient tells you something's not right, trust them—it's not.

Where are my helpers, you ask? There are only two, and one of them is giving a fevered patient a bed bath and the other one is changing the sheets for a patient with horrible diarrhea. The patient is so embarrassed and keeps apologizing, saying that no matter how hard she tries, she just can't make it to the bathroom in time.

Did I mention that on this same day, my daughter had a play at school? I put her in a private school so she'd be close to the hospital and maybe, just maybe, I could sometimes make it to her activities. I didn't make it that day. But it was amazing how my little seven-year-old daughter knew I worked at the hospital with sick people and seemed to understand that sometimes I just couldn't leave.

Let's recap the day. I have five patients. One is post-surgical and pain meds aren't working, one is being taken to surgery to repair his lung from a complication of his earlier procedure, one is throwing up, one is confused, and one just wants some water.

As my eight-hour shift comes to a close, I've somehow gotten everyone settled down. Charting is done, my manager needs to see me about something (I've finished my CEUs for my license, which is due to be renewed next month). But the shift is finally over. I talk to the manager, agree to change my schedule, clock out, and head down the stairs to go home to my daughter who, despite me not making it to her play, will be happy to see me.

But just as I turn the corner to go down the stairs, I remember that I never got my patient her water. I go back up the stairs, down to the kitchen area, get a cup of ice with water, fill a pitcher up with ice and water, and head down to the room. I apologize as I walk in, knowing there's nothing I can say, except that I'm sorry for not bringing her ice water. Her reply was, "Never mind; my husband got me some hours ago. You're a horrible nurse. I hope you're not my nurse tomorrow."

Oh, but I will be. I'll be back tomorrow, and I will probably have the same or a very similar set of patients, and I will do the best I can to take care of all of their needs and their families' needs, and I will probably miss my daughter's parent/teacher conference.

But that's okay, because I'm doing the absolute best that I can and today, when the confused lady finally understood no one was trying to get her, she looked at me with relief written all over her face and smiled and thanked me for being her angel and helping take care of the bad people who were trying to get her. She put her arms out for a hug, which I gladly gave her with a smile, because in that one moment, I knew I had made a difference.

You'll have days when you just can't seem to get everything done, and days when, as you go in each room, the patients seem to be sicker and sicker. There will be days when you can't catch a break and won't have time for a break—not a short break or a lunch break or a bathroom break. You'll go home and it'll seem like you've never been so tired. And you'll get up and go back the next time you're scheduled.

But each time, you'll have tried your best, and some days it's good enough and some days, for some patients, it won't be. And when you go home, in your head you may replay the day in a thousand ways, wishing you could have done it differently. But you gave it your best shot, and that's all anyone can ask of you. And it's all you can ask of yourself.

CHAPTER TWENTY-ONE

Touching the Lives of Strangers

Dear Kasey,

Some days are just going to be hard. There is no way to pre-pare you and nothing that I can say to you to help you through it. Horrible things happen to people; sometimes it's their own fault, sometimes it's just the universe. Do what you can to help, but try to never lose your faith in God, hu-mankind, and life. You will see horrible things, you will see amazing things, and you will make a difference.

Love, Aunt Kim

You'll see amazing things as a nurse. You'll see people survive when there's no rational explanation for how.

But mostly, you'll see a lot of sadness and death be-cause of things that could have been prevented if the patient had just done the right thing. Even if you work in Labor and Delivery, you'll have to face the issues of life and death. Some you'll agree with and some you won't. Some will cut you to the core and make you wish for a moment that you weren't a nurse. But mostly you'll make a small difference and touch the lives of people who are going through a horrible time in their life, and you'll be there to help them get through it.

That's what nursing is all about—not just helping people get better but helping them cope with the horrible realities of life. That's never why we go into nursing, to merely be with people in the most difficult times of their lives. We went into nursing to help people—you know, the "feel good" kind of help. But your life is about to change because more than any other career, you'll see things happen to people that change their lives and the lives of their family and friends forever. And I can assure you—it definitely does not feel good much of the time.

I've cared for so many patients. Here are some of the *hard* ones that immediately stick out in my memory:

A man who had been in a car wreck who we knew was probably the man who'd been running nurses off the road with his car, making them stop, and then raping them.

The patient who had shot and killed one of our police officers.

A man who had been beaten up by the father of a little girl the patient had been accused of molesting.

A man who was driving drunk and had hit another car, killing a family of five while he merely had a broken arm.

A child who had been shot by his dad "accidentally"— the dad had been playing Russian roulette with the gun while pointing it at the little kid's head.

A recruited football player who was killed because he wasn't wearing his seatbelt.

The mother and father of a fifteen-year-old boy, driving with them because he had just gotten his learner's permit. He wrecked, and both the mother and father were killed, leaving the four kids without parents. They were on their way from Texas to Disney for a family vacation.

The mother of a child who had been abused by the male members of her family to the point of needing surgery, and all the mother could say to me was that "she guessed she would have to put the child on birth control."

Too-many-to-count teenagers who were in car wrecks from drunk driving and died of head injuries, leaving their families devastated and questioning what they could have done differently. Or who had diving accidents while drunk and jumped into ponds, lakes, and springs that were too shallow and broke their neck, only to be paralyzed for the rest of their life due to one bad decision while drinking.

Countless AIDS patients who were dying alone because their parents had disowned them for being gay.

And motorcycle riders dying from wrecks who weren't wearing a helmet because they thought they'd be okay.

I think it's interesting that police officers, firefighters, paramedics, and first responders get a lot of credit for doing what they do, *as they should*. But does anyone think about the fact that when they save or rescue people, they take them to doctors and nurses? We work together to figure out a plan to help them and then the doctors move to the next patient.

The nurses are at the bedside for the duration of the recovery. We have to help them put the pieces back together—their bodies, their lives, the losses, and their new reality. We have to stand by them as they fight to heal all of that or help the family deal with the loss. Sometimes, I've wished I didn't have to go back to the ICU unit and deal with patients I knew wouldn't make it. I knew I'd have to be there for the family, and it's a horrible, hard situation. But every day we go back, not just on the days we are scheduled but the days to help out extra, because our patients and families need us. That's just what we as nurses do.

CHAPTER TWENTY-TWO

The Not-So-Fun Side of Nursing

Dear Kasey,

As I started writing this book, there were a million things I wanted to tell you. Things I wanted to prepare you for. Things they don't teach you in nursing school. In the previous chapters, I've tried to do that. This chapter will be different. This chapter will be about my frustrations and hurt and sometimes even the anger I've encountered over the years of being a nurse.

Love, Aunt Kim

You can't save all the patients, and sometimes, you lose the ones you shouldn't and also save the ones you shouldn't. We are not God; we can't make life and death decisions. All we can do is treat each patient the exact same way, put every bit of our knowledge, caring, and compassion into play for the patient in front of us. It doesn't matter if they are a murderer or rapist, or what they have or haven't done. They are first and foremost—and always—your patient.

Sometimes you'll end your shift and be so raging mad

that you can't see straight. And you know what—that's okay because that's all a part of being a nurse.

Some days people have complained—even while shouting at me—about what a lousy nurse I am because I took too long to get their meds, or their food, or to help them go to the restroom. Families get in on it as well, criticizing you for what you did or didn't do. I always felt like I should say something to them like, "I'm sorry," or, "I wish I could have done better." Or whatever words I can come up with to try to keep from feeling like I was apologizing for something when I didn't do anything wrong.

I can hold my bladder for over fourteen hours if I need to. I know I can go without food or water for over twelve hours and not even show I'm hungry or thirsty. I can pretend I'm just fine. I can smile and ask the next patient how they are feeling today and meet their kids knowing that I just missed my little girl's play today, the one she specifically asked me to be there for. I can wipe my tears dry from leaving the patient's family that just said goodbye to their thirty-something-year-old mother, and walk into the next room and act like I don't have anything else in the world to do but smile and meet the needs of this current patient and family.

I may be working a double shift, not because I want to but because one of the other nurses finally gave in to the fact that they have been sick for the past four days and is now at home recovering. Now she will probably be out for a week or more because she tried to do the right thing and come in to help out because she didn't want to leave us short. And also, it's possible she unintentionally passed her cold or flu to one of our coworkers, and they'll now need to be out.

The next room you enter may have someone who was told to be here at 5:30 a.m. for a 7:30 a.m. surgery. But before they got into surgery, the surgeon had an emergency case from the Emergency Room, and they got bumped. It's now almost noon, and the patient is tired of waiting and is hungry. If their surgery had started on time, they'd probably be getting ready to go home about now. And you catch all that frustration and anger because you're the one at the bedside.

You ask if they want you to see about rescheduling, and they get really upset. You completely understand and make the mistake of saying something like, "I'm just really glad it's not you in the emergency surgery," and boy, does that just make matters worse. You tried to think of the right thing to say, but guess what? There's no right thing to say.

Another favorite is working in the Recovery Room and there are no beds in the hospital. My patient had been out of surgery for over twenty-three hours and was ready to get to their room and see their family. I had let them talk to their family on the phone, but they wanted to see them. But family couldn't come into the Recovery Room due to the privacy of the other patients. That didn't go over well.

Neither did the fact that the only thing they could eat or drink was saltine crackers and water. They want something to *eat*. But you can't bring in hot, great-smelling food because the smell might make some of the other recovering patients sick. Again, not the patient's fault, and not your fault, but who is the patient and family getting upset with? You as the nurse.

What's even more fun is when you're the boss as well. They ask to speak to the head nurse or the nurse manager, and you have to tell them, "That's me, too." You would like to think they'd see that "all hands are on deck" trying to help with the overcrowded situation, but they only want to talk to the next higher-up person.

I get it. They have had their surgery scheduled for over three weeks; the hospital knew they were coming, so why wasn't a bed held for them? The true answer is that the Emergency Room was packed last night with a lot of admissions for the flu and some car accidents. All the beds got filled up. Still, this doesn't explain why at least one bed wasn't held. I guess they think it should be run like a hotel, with reservations. I can't say that's a bad idea, but the people who'd been waiting in the Emergency Room for eight hours, on a hard stretcher, were very glad when they finally got a bed. But again, you're at the bedside and you take the heat.

And sometimes you've taken all that you can. You're dealing with sick people, people in pain, families losing their loved ones, people who can't even get into a bed so they can eat and see their family; surgeons who are frustrated because if you can't get the Recovery Room clear, they can't start another surgery. Staff in the OR are stressed because they are ready to go with an open OR, but they can't use it because there's no bed. Meanwhile, the Emergency Department is overflowing and there's no stop gate. Sick people keep coming through their doors. People are waiting in the halls for beds. Administration is doing what they can, and many people are working extra shifts and overtime and coming in on their days off to help. It's not for lack of trying. There are just too many damn sick people and absolutely nothing you can do.

You're tired, frustrated, angry, hungry, and need to pee, but there just isn't time. And I'd like to tell you that this type of day happens once a month. But honestly, it probably happens at least once a week, if not more often, depending on the season.

And let's not forget about full moons and the havoc they can wreak, with lots of babies being born, more people heading to the hospital, and people acting more stupid than usual. Yes, it's true; many nurses do follow the lunar schedule so they can request time off—or at least be prepared—for days when there's a full moon.

As I write this, I'm not angry or disappointed in my career choice. I don't wish I had chosen another career path. I'm just telling you what real nursing looks like.

There are definitely two different sides to every story. And here is the other side of nursing.

You're at the bedside of a patient who everyone thought wouldn't make it, and you see the look on his mama's face when he squeezes her hand on command even though he has a machine breathing for him. When a patient has a head injury, you give them a "command" to make sure they're actually interacting. A reaction is different than a reflex. For example, "squeeze my hand" confirms they understand. They're not just responding. They're intentionally responding.

Or the patient wakes up after surgery and the doctor comes in to tell them and their family that they eliminated all the cancer and it looked like everything will be okay.

Or you hear your name called from down the hall and,

as you turn around, the patient you took care of this morning is staring at you. He calls out to anyone listening, "Just wanted to say goodbye to my favorite nurse."

Or watching a baby being born, seeing a new human being for the first time and realizing that life does go on and that it'll work out and be okay. And yes, eventually you'll get to go to the bathroom, or get something to eat, or better yet, you'll get to go home and see your own family.

The good outweighs the bad. You just need to make sure you drill the good memories into your mind so you can call on them during the bad times. Because sometimes it feels like the bad times outweigh the good times. But overall, I'd say that with all the good and bad, a nursing career is worth it. You did your best and did what you could to help the patient and their family in their time of crisis. And sometimes you're the only one who will ever tell yourself that. But believe it, because as a nurse, you're making a difference. You're caring and compassionate, and the job is worth it. And if amazing people like you didn't do it, who would?

CHAPTER TWENTY-THREE

Making the Tough Decisions

Dear Kasey,

There will be more policy and procedures and guidelines in your job than you'll ever be able to read. To me, policy and procedures are based on basic rules and a lot of common sense. But don't ever let a piece of paper hold you back from doing the right thing for your patient. I'm not telling you to break the rules. I'm asking you to do what you think needs to be done for your patient. Follow your policy and procedures, teaching, and experience but most of all follow your gut. It'll never lead you wrong.

Love, Aunt Kim

We all get frustrated with our jobs but being a nurse makes it interesting. In most jobs, if you lose it and spout off, it's to your coworkers and in a private space away from clients. But nurses are often in the patient's room. You're tired and "the patient is always right." And I agree with that statement, but seriously, sometimes the patients has a skewed perception of the situation. One patient woke up in the recovery room and said she hadn't gotten *any* pain meds for the two hours she was there. I was the Nurse Manager at the time, and the nurse had called me to the bedside to let me know what was going on. I had seen the patient get meds and knew that she was medicated. I thought that when she woke up some more, she'd remember.

That didn't happen. She was even more upset when she got up on the floor. She complained and I was called to the room. I could say nothing to convince her that she had gotten meds. She claimed that the nurse was using the meds herself and giving her fake meds. It was ridiculous, *and* she demanded that I fire the nurse. I wanted to defend my nurse, but I couldn't because there was no convincing the patient. So we took the hit. I said I'd take care of it, and that's how it ended. Interestingly enough, the patient thought I meant I was firing the nurse. That was the only thing that would make her happy. Needless to say, I didn't fire the nurse, and I didn't lie to the patient, but it was very frustrating since "we" had done nothing wrong.

I smile when I think about how we're often referred to as angels. If you could read our minds, sometimes you'd see that we're anything but angels. We have feelings and get frustrated and angry and upset and disappointed, and, sometimes, it gets away from us—*but* very rarely. We aren't angels because we are human, and as humans, we can only take so much.

Let's talk about some more negative things about nursing—the diseases you can catch. What other role (other than, perhaps, being a scientist with the CDC) knowingly and sometimes unknowingly exposes you to life-threatening diseases? Not to mention dangerous patients who are confused and disoriented and very strong due to the medications they're on. For some reason, super-confused little old people can fight back with amazing strength.

When I started my career, AIDS was just beginning to show itself and so many people were dying of it. Now, we've gotten a grip on the disease, and so many people live with AIDS that it's no longer a death sentence.

There have been many little diseases and we started using too many antibiotics, so suddenly we then got all these new antibiotic-resistant infections. Now we have MRSA and necrotizing fasciitis (NF). They are amazingly resistant diseases, and NF is a horrible, horrible disease process that causes so many losses of limbs and life. Then there are the diabetic foot ulcers and the issue with vascular circulation, and the MRSA seems to jump on any wound and make a nightmare out of it.

Yes, we use gloves, gowns, masks, and all the appropriate protective gear, but then it's so hard to care for patients. Starting an IV with gloves on is a little crazy. The person is already so sick, and then you add the fact that they have had strong antibiotics and medications through their IV and it becomes difficult to get an IV site. PICC lines have made a great difference, but there are still so many challenges.

How can a patient sit in the waiting room with no isolation precautions and now, suddenly, they're in a private room and even if we just walk into the room, we need to gear up? I know we obviously need to put on protective gear for some things, but sometimes, it seems the precautions put us more at risk because of the awkwardness.

Now let's talk about regulations. *Are you kidding me?*

Back in the day, we had policies and procedures to follow. If it was a policy or procedure, then there was no exception to the rule—*it must be followed as it was written.* Now we have advanced to guidelines, which I think are wonderful for the most part. Guidelines are just that: they are there to help you with most situations, but it ultimately comes down to using good judgment, knowledge, and experience, and doing what needs to be done. However, you still just need to use common sense for so many things—*instead* of merely following a rule.

As a Nurse Manager, I told my staff that if they made a decision in the best interest of the patient and could explain why they did what they did, then I'd back them up. Nursing isn't always about following policies and guidelines; it's about doing what's best for the patient. And that can mean so many different things. Please don't look for reasons to break policy or guidelines, but when it comes down to it, *don't* let policies and guidelines stop you from doing what's best for your patient.

These days, dogs (or other animals) are allowed in the hospital as therapy dogs. But years ago, it wasn't considered a good idea. One of my patients in ICU was dying and couldn't go home and say goodbye to her little dog. That was all she wanted. I knew it was important to her, so some of the staff and I devised a plan to sneak the little dog in and let the patient say goodbye. It was one of the smartest things I've ever done. The look on the lady's face when she saw her dog was priceless. To see her smiling around her breathing tube and reaching up to hold the little dog was a sight I will never forget. Did I break a policy? Yes. Was it in the best interest of the patient? Yes. Would

I do it again? Absolutely! We let the dog stay for about fifteen minutes and then took it back home. The lady died later that night. I swear she had a smile on her face.

A wonderful chief of nursing once taught me a valuable lesson. She said, "Sometimes it's better to beg for forgiveness than to ask for permission. If you can always say yes to the question, "Was it in the best interest of the patient?" then you can stand up to any board or judge and support your decision. That's important. Make sure you keep your priorities straight—that you're indeed doing it for the best interest of your patient—and you can never go wrong.

CHAPTER TWENTY-FOUR

Quads

Dear Kasey,

You will see lots of things in your career that aren't fair and shouldn't have happened. Welcome to the world of nursing. You're trying to do what you can and make a difference. You won't always see the difference; you just have to go with "I did the best I could." Some things you just can't change.

Love, Aunt Kim

I can think of a lot of things that happen to our patients and families, but for me, a patient who has become a quad (short for quadriplegic) is probably the worst. I remember a twenty-year-old college kid who dove out of a boat because all his other friends were doing it. But he hit a stump and was instantly paralyzed from the neck down. He couldn't even breathe for himself, but one of his buddies knew CPR, so he breathed for him until the EMS team could get there. This kid had his whole life in front of him. He was in college, had lots of friends, and had a supportive girlfriend. None of that changed, yet everything changed—so much was taken away, within mere seconds. I'm not saying someone who's a quad can't go on and live a very full life, do amazing things, and be a great role model. I'm only saying that in one minute, their life changes. Then they have to learn who they really are and what they really want out of life—because their plans have changed completely.

Someone must feed them and bathe them; a machine breathes for them; nurses, doctors, and all sorts of staff care for them. They can't do anything. Even if they can breathe, the only thing they can do is talk and turn their head.

Early in my career, one of my patients was a quad. It taught me so much and is probably one of the hardest memories I have. Her life was affected and changed forever, but unknown to me at the time, it would forever change me and my life as well.

Annie. She was an eighty-plus-year-old woman in very good health who was riding with someone else when they got into a little fender-bender. But that jerk was enough to snap her head and neck, causing her second cervical to tear her spinal cord and make her completely paralyzed, unable even to breathe for herself.

I worked the night shift at this time, and I took care of Annie from the first night until she was moved from the unit. I'd go into her room, give her medications, turn and position her, feed her, clean her up, talk to her, and do whatever other daily living activities she needed. Think about the fact that she couldn't brush her own teeth or hair; she couldn't feed herself; she couldn't wipe herself; she couldn't do anything.

After a short time, when they realized her paralysis was permanent, they put in a trach (a hole in her neck) so she could at least talk for short periods of time over the breathing machine. I enjoyed talking with Annie and asking her about her children, grandchildren, her husband, her life, and everything and anything I could think of. I'd ask questions and see if I could get her talking, because sometimes it's hard for them to discuss what they are really feeling, but if you can get them started, sometimes the true feelings come up and you can try to help. Most of the time, you're just talking to them because it's too hard for them to try to talk. But some nights she was up to it, and she would share some of her story.

She had led an amazing, happy life. I loved hearing all her stories. This sounds like a conversation that any nurse could be having with any of their patients at the end of their life, but let me explain it in a little more detail. In order for Annie to talk, you would *remove the breathing tube from her trachea*, and she'd talk until she ran out of breath. Then you would put the vent tube back on her trach so she could get her breath, after which she could get a few more sentences out. A simple two- to three-minute conversation took ten to fifteen minutes because you had to allow time for the vent to breathe for her. It was a struggle for her, and talking wore her out, but she seemed to have a lot that she wanted to say.

One night during one of our conversations, she looked up at my face, made eye contact with me, and tilted her head down toward her trach. That was her signal that she wanted me to take the tube off the trach so she could talk. I will never forget her words that night.

She said, "I've lived a wonderful, amazing life, and I'm ready to go. I don't want to live this way, and I want you to turn off the breathing machine and just let me go."

I said, "Annie, I can't do that."

She asked why not, and I didn't have an answer for her. I just put her trach tube back on.

That was all we said that night, but the next time I walked into the room, she nodded toward her trach. I removed it and she said, "My name is Annie Smith. I'm of sound mind and body, and I understand that if you remove this breathing machine, I will stop breathing and die. I want you to leave it off and not put it back on."

I tried not to cry as I placed the trach tube back on.

All my life I've had animals who I love. Some people see their animals as family, not just pets, and it's horrible when you lose them or, worse yet, make the decision to put them to sleep or let them go due to their health. I could do that for them, but I could do nothing for Annie.

Lying before me was an eighty-year-old woman who was telling me that she had led a wonderful life but didn't want to spend any more time having to be completely cared for and dependent on everyone and everything— just so she could lie around in a bed all the time, unable to do anything for herself. She was asking me to let her die. She never asked me outright to kill her, but that was essentially what she was doing. I had no legal right to do that; no one in the medical community could help her. There were no laws.

We explained to her that the only way she could be taken off the vent was if she could breathe on her own or if her heart stopped. The next thing we knew, she was asking us to help her "practice" breathing. She thought if she could build her shoulder muscles up enough, she could at least pretend to breathe, and we could take the tube off. She practiced and practiced and practiced, but her muscles had atrophied since the injury. There was no way she could build them back up, but we tried.

It became a very bad situation. We cared for Annie and did everything she needed, but not the one thing she wanted. She got to the point that when you walked into her room, she'd motion toward her trach, and when you removed it so she could talk, she'd repeat the same thing over and over and over again: "My name is Annie. I'm of sound mind and body, and I want you to take me off this machine so I can die."

After about a month, she was transferred to a long-term facility that could take her on the vent. This wonderfully sweet woman, who had led a fulfilling life, was sent out of our unit to a place that didn't know her. Where she'd have to learn to interact with new people, and they'd have to learn her needs. But I guess, in the long run, it wouldn't matter where she went—no one would be able to do the only thing she asked of us.

I didn't keep up with her or learn of what happened to her. I couldn't. I've always felt bad about not continuing to check on her, but I emotionally couldn't handle it. And there were others to care for and cry over. Her suffering wasn't mine to carry.

Her family was very supportive of anything that she wanted, but there was nothing they could do. They'd come and visit and talk to her and cry with her and for her. There was nothing any of us could do.

I don't know what I want you to learn from this story. Maybe after all this time, I just needed to put it in writing. Did I feel like I failed her? Could I have done something different? Should I have helped her? It doesn't matter what the answer to any of those questions is, because this happened so long ago.

I guess I wanted you to know one of the saddest situations I've ever found myself in with a patient. At some point, no matter what area you choose, you'll have an Annie patient. And you'll do what you need to do, and no matter what, it'll be okay. Even though it doesn't feel okay.

Remember that as nurses, we see people at their weakest, most vulnerable, and saddest times in their life. You must put your personal feelings aside and do what is best for the patient.

You, as a newbie nurse, will have moments in your career when you will doubt yourself and whether or not you did all you could. You might consider yourself a failure and second-guess yourself. That is just part of the job. It is human nature to second-guess your actions even though you made them years ago regarding a certain patient. Once the hard work is done, you must make sure you take care of yourself.

Nursing can be hard and sad and challenging and difficult and confusing and frustrating and so many things. And even though it doesn't feel like it much of the time, you *will* be okay.

CHAPTER TWENTY-FIVE

Nurse or Family

Dear Kasey,

This is one of the hardest chapters to write. But I want you to know about it because one day, you too may be in a position where you have to be family and nurse. It's not easy. I kept trying to make myself stay in either the daughter role or the nurse role, but you can't separate the two. That's who you are now, and I'm so proud of you.

Love, Aunt Kim

One of the most horrible—yet most amazing—moments for me as a nurse was being at the bedside of my own daddy at his time of death. I don't know why I want to talk to you about it, but I do. For now, we will cover the events leading up to his death. I'll discuss his actual death later.

I received a call from my mama telling me that Daddy was having problems breathing and that they were at the ER two hours away from me. I quickly handled whatever needed to be handled and left within minutes to go see what was going on.

While I was getting ready to go, the conversation I had with my daddy about eight weeks ago came rushing back into my mind. I kept replaying it over and over on the two-hour drive to see him.

Daddy was sixty-four-years old and had been a severe diabetic since about the age of thirty-nine. The years of the disease had caused quite a bit of kidney damage, but they were still working. I talked to him about having dialysis if the diabetes took out his kidneys. He told me he had watched his friends' lives be taken over by dialysis and he didn't want to live that way. He'd rather just go ahead and go.

Those next three days are a blur. I remember some things, but I don't remember everything in the order it happened. When I arrived at the hospital, he was already in his room. I remember being told he'd had a heart attack and that it had damaged his kidneys. I remember talking to him about letting us put him on dialysis. And he again said he really didn't want to have dialysis—the same thing he'd told me a few weeks ago. As a nurse, I knew that dialysis would help him, but I remembered the conversation, and honoring someone's wishes is very important as a nurse.

As a daughter, I didn't want to lose my daddy, but the nursing side of me realized that's what was happening. If you need dialysis and you choose not to do it, it's only a matter of time before your electrolytes get unbalanced and take you out.

I had seen my daddy's numbers and knew that he wouldn't last long without dialysis. By "not long," I mean days or hours. I went to his bedside and asked him to please consider dialysis for me. I don't know if that was fair or not, but it's what I did. I wanted some time. He asked if he started it, would he have the option to stop it. I assured him he would, and I even told him—*promised* him—that if the staff at the hospital wouldn't remove the tubes, I would. And I would have. Removing dialysis tubes isn't within the practice of an RN, but it wouldn't have mattered. I'd have done it anyway.

He agreed, and he and Mama were quickly taken to the dialysis unit, a dual line was placed in his right groin, and dialysis was started. It can take up to about four hours, and the doctor told me he wanted to try to remove at least two liters from my dad.

After about an hour, they wheeled Daddy out, and the minute I saw him, I knew dialysis had not helped and had been the wrong decision. He looked horrible and was throwing up. Mama was there right by his side, and he was wheeled back to his room and put into his bed. The doctor asked him if we could leave them in place for the night and possibly try again in the morning. Daddy agreed, even knowing he'd need to keep that right leg straight all night. But he said that was fine.

Looking back, I regret asking him to do it, but at the time, the daughter part of me took over. I didn't want to lose my daddy.

That night was truly the longest night of my life. Because they couldn't get the fluid off of him, and because he had to lie down the entire time due to the arterial lines in his groin, his lungs started filling up with fluid. Mama and I were with him the whole time. Every thirty to forty minutes or so, we could tell he was getting confused, but the minute he sat up, his mind would clear. We would remind him that he couldn't get up, and he was very amicable. Completely with it. I was too distraught as his daughter to be able to look at the entire picture. All I knew was that I didn't want him to bleed out from his groin since I was the one who had talked him into getting the tubes in the first place.

He'd sit up, and I'd remind him to keep his leg straight. We tried restraining his leg to help "remind" him about keeping it straight, but each time, after thirty minutes or so, he'd get confused and get up. Mama and I tried to keep him in bed but couldn't. I was so scared that the tubes would puncture his artery and he'd bleed out. The only time he wasn't confused was when he was sitting up, which was the only thing he couldn't do. He was strong enough to sit up, but it was dangerous because of his tube.

Those of you with experience, or who have dealt with this in clinical already, probably already see the problem. He was going into congestive heart failure. When he'd lay down, the fluids would be all over his lungs, which would drop his O2 saturation, which would then make him confused, so he'd try to sit up so he could breathe. Then he'd clear, understand that he needed to keep his leg straight, and lay back down. It was a vicious cycle.

This next part will probably be one of the hardest things I've ever had to write about, and as a nurse, one of the hardest things I've had to witness.

We weren't in my hospital. I was out of my element in knowing who to call for help. My daddy was the patient, and I was so upset about the massive heart attack that I was thinking about losing him as a daughter, not analyzing him as a patient.

I kept going to our nurse, telling him that Daddy was getting up and wouldn't stay flat and that I thought something was going on. He'd come to the room, help us get him back in bed, and tell Daddy he needed to lie flat because of the tubes. Daddy would say he understood but that sometimes he just had to get up. The nurse had come on at 7 p.m. and was working till 7 a.m., so he was with us through the night as Daddy kept going through the cycle of lying down, getting confused, getting up, and being put back to bed. I went out to tell the nurse that Daddy was up again and tried to talk to him about what he thought was going on. He asked if I was thinking like a daughter or like a nurse. That stumped me. I was trying to do both. It wasn't making sense that he cleared up when he got up, yet was so confused after lying down for a while. But I wasn't sure I was thinking right, so I followed the nurse back into the room, where my daddy was standing at the foot of the bed.

The nurse grabbed my daddy by the gown and threw him backwards into bed and said, "I'm too busy for this tonight; you need to stay in bed and quit being such a problem." I was done. Let's just say my daughter and nurse modes both kicked into overdrive, and when that son of a bitch turned around, I said in a level, even tone, "You just fucked up." Then I told him to get out of our room, get his charge nurse in the room, have someone call his nurse manager, and get me a doctor in the room *now*. By the time I got to the word *now*, I'm sure I was screaming. I've never been so mad in my life. Daughter, nurse, human, whatever—*no one should ever be treated that way*, and certainly not my daddy.

I never laid a hand on him; I was afraid to because of what I might do. I'm a country girl, and you don't mess with us. You damn sure didn't mess with my Daddy. I stepped back so he could leave the room, and in about five minutes, ten or more people were in the room—one of them being the charge nurse. I informed her that the nurse was never to be allowed in our room again for any reason.

Now that we had everyone's attention, they wanted to put my daddy on a vent and emergency dialysis him. Three ER doctors were in the room, but I realized that if Daddy didn't want to be on dialysis, he certainly wouldn't want to wake up and find out that he was on a breathing machine.

At this point, my daddy was semi-comatose. I asked them to call his personal doctor at home because I knew he'd come help us with the shape Daddy was in—dying.

It didn't take him long to get to us. He talked to me first and told me that my daddy's ejection fraction was less than ten percent, and that his kidneys were definitely in failure. He didn't think they'd recover from the damage that had been done to the heart.

He was silent for a few minutes, then put his hand on my shoulder and asked if I remembered the conversation we'd had two months prior with Daddy. I told him I did and asked if he thought Daddy would just want us to keep him comfortable and let the family stay with him instead of intubating him and transferring him to the ICU, where we could only visit for ten minutes on the hour. We agreed that keeping him comfortable with the family was the better option for our situation and discussed it with the rest of the family.

But let's talk about that nurse for a minute. I know he was busy and that my daddy was turning out to be a very high-maintenance patient. In hindsight, we now know he was acting that way because he was going into organ failure; he was dying. Yet that nurse wouldn't listen to me, humiliated me by asking the "nurse/daughter" question, and didn't read the signs or try to help us. He failed to meet the needs of anyone.

I've often wondered whether, if he had analyzed things early in the shift, around 7 or 8 p.m., he could have caught what was going on soon enough to lead to a different outcome. No, I don't think it would have kept my daddy from dying, but what a difference he could have made in our lives while we were losing someone so important to us. He shouldn't have talked to me as a nurse; I was stressed out, and my daddy was lying in that bed. He wasn't just some patient—he was one of the most important people in the world to me. That nurse had no compassion for me or any of our family. But most importantly, he failed as a nurse to the one person who was so important: the patient, my daddy.

This experience was so raw and emotional for me—devastating and enraging. And honestly, I don't have grand lessons I want you to learn from my heart wrenching experience. I mostly just wanted to share that I know what it's like to be on the other side.

In that moment, there were so many things that could have and should have been done differently. But I can't do anything about it now. I can only hope that maybe you will read this and try to keep in mind that so many of your patients are deeply suffering—and that compassion goes a long way.

You'll be pushed to the very edge of your sanity for a variety of reasons. But please always remember that the patient is sick and in the hospital for a reason and you're there to try to help. Try to keep their humanity in perspective as you do the best you can.

CHAPTER TWENTY-SIX

It Still Matters

Dear Kasey,

As I write down my memories and experiences to help you with your career, it seems that once I remember one patient, that memory alone then brings back so many more. We all have our individual morals and values, and you'll meet people, both as professionals and patients and families, whose values are so different from yours. My suggestion is that it's important to listen to them. I promise you'll learn something; it might not change your own opinion, but it'll help you see things from a lot of different views. That's not just about being a nurse; that's about being a human being.

Love, Aunt Kim

In your nursing class at school, there was a wide variety of people—women and men, young and old. Some you had lots in common with, some not so much. Everyone is raised in their own unique ways and has developed their own beliefs based on how they were raised or through their individual experiences.

You'll experience some things as a nurse that go against your personal beliefs. For example, if a twelve-year-old girl comes in pregnant from abuse, and the family has decided on an abortion, you have to care for her and support the family in their care of her.

Do you think you agree with euthanasia, or are you absolutely sure you don't believe in it? It's very much an individual answer to an extremely difficult question. I've only considered it on one patient in my career, Annie, whom I told you about earlier. But one thing you'll learn as a nurse is that life decisions are not always as cut and dry as you'd like to think. You'll see things, experience things, and feel things that will confuse you, and you won't know what you need to do, are doing, or should do. And that's okay. Sometimes your answer will be different depending on the circumstances.

Now consider an eighty-six-year-old man who's had a massive stroke, is in a coma, and has extensive brain damage proven by a CT scan of the head. You've been the main nurse, and the family has indicated they just want to let the patient go peacefully. You come in for your shift the next day, and the patient is still there. The family has decided to keep the patient on the ventilator, add a feeding tube, and keep the patient as a full code. *What?* You sat with them yesterday and supported them when the doctor told them there was no hope. What happened? What changed their mind?

It doesn't matter. They've changed their mind, and you have to be just as supportive today about keeping him alive as you were yesterday about letting him go.

As nurses, we are in such an important position in the eyes of patients and families, so be very careful about what you say and who you say it to. They're looking to us for answers that sometimes we just don't have. And even if we do, we don't need anyone making decisions based on what we think. It has to be the patient and their family's decisions.

I've tried to help patients and families by making sure they understand what they've been told and that they understand their options, but I've always tried to make sure I in no way influenced their decision. The last thing in the world you want is for someone to make a decision based on what you told them and then they regret it and think it's your fault. You can help them understand their options, but you can never make their decisions for them. That's their burden and theirs alone to make and live with.

Children, for me, are the hardest. The amazing thing is that they are so resilient. You never really know how amazing their little body is, and it's hard to know what will happen. We think the answer about life support is so much easier when it's an older person who has led an amazing, relatively long life. But that about when it's a five-year-old laying on that bed, a child who should have his whole life in front of him, and the family has to decide how much is too much brain damage and what the right decision is? The fact that he was drowning because no one was watching him adds all sorts of emotion to the situation. You don't even have to have your own children for this to be a heart-wrenching situation.

You won't have all the answers; you can't have all the answers. You're human and will have feelings. Sometimes family members argue with each other about what needs to happen or "what Daddy would want," or they want to just give him a little more time. We think we know what we would do if it was our decision to make, but trust me, it's never, ever an easy decision.

It never gets easier. The situations I address now, at the end of my career, are no easier to deal with than they were for me as a newbie nurse. When I think about this, I'm glad it hasn't changed. I still do really care about my patients. After all, I'm a nurse, and maybe, just maybe, there's a little of that angel still in me. And I know you have that angel in you.

CHAPTER TWENTY-SEVEN

Angels or Bitches

Dear Kasey,

Try to remember that, to me, you'll always be an angel!

Love, Aunt Kim

It seems nurses are seen either as angels or non-caring bitches. I've been putting off writing this conclusion for a variety of reasons. Truth be told, I cringe when I hear people call nurses angels. I can only speak for myself, but I know that in no way am I an angel. As I let my mind drift back over my years as a nurse, a lot comes to mind that isn't pretty. If you could see what I've seen, had to do some of the things I've done, and thought some of the things I've thought, I doubt you'd think you were an angel, either. At most, I could possibly be from one of those songs about angels with broken wings.

People say, "Ah, but the profession you've chosen is one of caring for others." Yes, that's true. But more than anything else, as we draw this book to a close, I want you to remember: we are human; we make mistakes; we get tired; we get hurt; sometimes we get angry, and, yes, sometimes we say things out loud that we shouldn't say. Don't even get me started on the things that run through our mind and shouldn't. Hence, broken wings.

I want to have written you a happy book. I want you to laugh. I want to give you a heads up on some things. I want you to know more than I knew going into this career. I want to protect you, and I want to help you. Perhaps most importantly, I want you to know this career is very hard but rewarding. You may find yourself having a very sad day, yet something or someone turns it into one of your best days ever. At the lowest point in your career, something or someone will restore your belief in what you're doing.

Believe me, though, most days are just about going to work, smiling, doing what you can, keeping that inner voice quiet, and making it to the end of your shift.

Your inner voice will ask things like, *"Am I the only one who cares about keeping things clean around here? Can she not hear herself and how awful she sounds? Does he not know that I don't want to hear about how everything has just been so easy for him as a nurse because he just flew through everything? Can't they, for just one day, not complain about the nurse manager, or how short-staffed we are, or how the hospital food is so lousy, or that they didn't get a lunch? For just one shift this month—hell, for just one hour this week—can they just quit complaining?"*

Everyone talks about all the angels in nursing, but frankly, I don't see them, much less act or think like one.

Why, you ask? Because we are overworked and under-paid, don't get breaks, may not get lunch, and deal with people who are mad at the world and want someone to take it out on. We clean poop, we hold people down to start an IV, we make people cry, and we hurt people just trying to change their dressings, all so they'll get better. We give them medicines that make them vomit, we give baths, and we get yelled at by others because of something we've done or haven't done. We aren't getting the patients ready for surgery fast enough; we aren't charting cor-rectly; we aren't charting enough. We aren't doing what we're supposed to be doing—and they wonder why we left our halo and wings at home.

I've been fortunate in my career to have worked at a variety of levels of nursing. I started out as a nursing as-sistant, then was a nurse tech, nursing student, graduate nurse, new nurse, assistant nurse manager, and nurse man-ager or director. I've had the amazing experience of being in a lot of different shoes, which has really helped me in my career. Now when I ask you to do something, I know what it's like to be where you are and can sympathize and empathize accordingly. However, sometimes, because I've been where you've been, all I want you to do right now is just do what I ask. I don't have time to explain, or ask you about your day, or ask you if you *can* do it. I just need you to do it.

I've had the privilege and honor of working in some amazing units with some amazing nurses and other staff members. There are a lot of great people out there. But health care is a hard field. It doesn't matter what level you're at or what position you're in—I know it's hard.

Yes, we have help. Respiratory therapists help with the ventilator; patient care assistants help with Foleys and baths; physical therapy helps with movement; pharmacy helps with medication; dietary brings us tube feedings. Secretaries answer the phone, call doctors, talk to families, and get us more of the paperwork we need. Charge nurses check in on us; other staff nurses come to help us catch up if they have somehow, miraculously, caught up themselves.

But when all is said and done, everything comes back to the nurse assigned to that patient for that shift. That nurse is the captain of the ship. No, it isn't the doctors. They come in and write orders, and they are very much a part of the team. But make no mistake about it, the captain of the ~~ship~~ shift is the nurse. Now that you're on the floor, working in this brave new world, you're the captain, too. Everything revolves around you and the decisions you make for your patient.

Let me "jump ship" here for a minute and say that if some adverse event happens to this patient, it doesn't matter who did what. You'll be the one interviewed by the lawyers and risk managers. No matter what happened, you'll be asked to answer for it. The wrong medication got ordered by the physician, and you gave it—it's on you. Pharmacy sent up the wrong medication, and you gave it—it's on you. Physical therapy didn't know the patient was on quiet time and turned on the lights and did their physical therapy session as ordered—it's on you.

The unit secretary let the patient's family in to see the patient. They asked you, but there was a misunderstanding because respiratory was asking at the same time about suctioning the patient and you said yes. The family has walked in while the patient is being suctioned, and they have now seen things they can't unsee—that's on you.

It's seven hours into your shift. You haven't eaten, peed, or taken a break. You've had nothing to drink; you forgot to call at 10 a.m. to get the information for your kid's trip. You forgot to arrange for someone to pick up that kid, and there's no way you'll make it out of here on time.

The family asked two hours ago about speaking to you about something they didn't like. Don't they understand you're doing everything you possibly can to keep their family member alive and don't have time for the questions?

You chose this career to make a difference. You chose the caring and compassionate career of taking care of others. Sometimes you sacrifice yourself, your family, and your friends for the needs of your patient and their family. And what do you get for it? Nothing. Oh, yeah, you get your salary, but some days no wage per hour will make your shift worth it. You'll want to quit and walk out and never come back.

You're finally finished for the day. You're going home two hours after your shift ended. You're exhausted, you haven't eaten, you still haven't peed, and you have no idea where your kid is. But as you leave, you have to pass by the waiting room, and unbelievably (cue eyeroll), your patient's family wants to talk to you. You cringe and think, "*I just want to go home,* and *I'm already clocked out.*" That inside voice is going crazy and says a lot of things it shouldn't be saying right now, but thankfully, those words stay inside.

You force yourself to smile and ask what they need. They tell you they just want to say thank you and tell you what an amazing angel you are. You thank them and turn to leave. They ask, "Please tell us that you'll be back tomorrow and will be our nurse again?"

You straighten your crooked halo that got knocked sideways when you hit your head on the monitor and pull your wings back up on your back. You smile, hug them, and say, "Of course I will be. I'll always be here for you."

And that, my dear, is what being a nurse is all about.

CONCLUSION

Dear Nurse

I don't think I can call this book complete without adding one more chapter, about the current crisis that we in nursing, and the entire world, are facing.

When I graduated in 1984, the AIDS epidemic was hitting the world. We knew nothing about it and were all scared that we were "going to catch it," because no one knew anything. And now, as you are entering the world of nursing, here comes the COVID-19 virus. Full-blown worldwide pandemic. What the hell? It is interesting—me being in the middle of the AIDS epidemic (at least, that is what they were calling it then) as a newbie nurse, and now, as an experienced RN at the end of my career, being in the middle of this pandemic.

I want you to know that it's going to be all right. I'm not saying this to keep you from being scared. I'm not saying it to try to calm you down. I'm not saying it to bullshit you. In nursing, you are going to face all sorts of

crises—things that will come and go. And you're going to
be just fine.

For you, at the beginning of your nursing career, the
world has turned upside down. The COVID-19 virus is
here. Emotions, opinions, and attitudes are all over the
place. Some people are ignoring the situation. Some people are holed up at home, scared of getting it. And the
nurses—well, the nurses are just doing their thing.

As I am typing this, our hospital with over seven hun-
dred beds is currently sitting at about 50-percent
occupancy. The Newborn ICU nursery census is down.
The ICU census is down. The floor occupancy is down.
And there are fewer than ten people in the hospital with
COVID-19 virus.

Things change daily. Some of the hospital staff aren't
getting their full hours, so they are being used to help
monitor the entries for employees, patients, and families.
Last week, if you were sick in the hospital, you could not
have a visitor with you. This week, if you are having surgery, you can't have someone with you, but if you spend
the night in the hospital, you can have one designated person.

There are people all over the country who are in ICU
beds, very sick and possibly dying, but we can't let their
family in to be with them because of the risk of spreading
the virus even more.

Back in the day of AIDS, we finally figured out how to
handle the epidemic. I think it's going to be a while before
we figure out this COVID thing. Right now, with COVID,
the only answer is that the world is wearing masks and
trying to practice social distancing. However, it seems that

it isn't real to people until someone they know has it. And folks, after that ... it's too late.

I think that soon, we will know a lot more about the spread of this virus. It's true that most people will get it and survive. The problem is that we really don't know who will do okay with it and who will die. And we certainly know that our elderly population is at risk, as well as people with significant health issues. But no matter how careful we all are, sometimes we are exposing ourselves and each other without even knowing it.

We are all over wearing the masks. We are all over people being sick. We are all over family not being together—and I think one of the biggest things is the fact that we are all over not being able to hug our family and friends. It's a big adjustment. We don't like it. Yet we remain in the middle of a worldwide health care crisis.

Thankfully, people did help turn the curve, but I think some people don't understand that when you turn the curve, that simply allows us in health care to take care of who is sick—because fewer people are getting sick at the same time. The overall number of people who are going to get the virus has not changed; its spread is just delayed, allowing us to have the room to care for everyone as they get it.

I have no answers or great words of wisdom to give you. I only want to say: this too shall pass.

As nurses, we are exposed to a lot of different things, and a lot of different diseases have come during my career—AIDS, MRSA, necrotizing fasciitis, C-Diff, and a lot of other diseases and infections that we don't really know about or understand. For you, there are even more ahead.

I think that because of how much we are exposed, our immune system is stronger. I think that because we know our co-workers and sick people are depending on us, we tough it out and go to work, even when we should be staying home. You just don't see the people in health care getting it at the same rate as the rest of the population. I can't prove or explain it definitively, but it seems to be true.

I have tried to tell you about nursing through this book, but there are so many more questions than answers. What matters is that you are out there helping us, trying to make a difference and doing the best you can. That's all anyone can ask of you, and it's all you can ask of yourself.

You have an amazing career ahead of you. It's going to be exciting and challenging. Just remember, when you have finally finished your shift for the day and are getting ready to go home, don't forget to straighten your halo and make sure your wings are on straight.

Thanks for being one of us.

Kim R. Edwards RN

APPENDIX

A Nurse Is...

Dear Kasey,

I want this to be a simple section about a few things that complete that sentence. I smile because every time I think about it, I add a few more things. I think if I could only use one word to complete that statement, it would be:

*"A nurse is **amazing**."*

Love, Aunt Kim

So you've almost finished nursing school, or have already finished, and are getting ready to start the wonderful career of *nursing*.

The very word *nurse* conjures up so many different feelings and emotions in everyone. And I mean everyone.

I've seen grown men cry talking about the nurse who took care of their wife as she was dying, and they refer to the nurse as an angel.

I've seen moms and dads with their new baby talking about how wonderful their labor and delivery nurse was (and no, that wasn't and will never be me), or maybe how wonderful the nurse taking care of their baby was.

I've heard people complaining about how lazy their nurse was and that they couldn't get help to the bathroom, get their linens changed, or get water.

The word *nurse* means so many different things to so many different people, but what does it mean to you? You're the *nurse*. You've gone through school, maybe even taken and passed boards (yes, you'll pass them), or perhaps started your first job.

At this point, on the backside of my career, I've thought a lot over many years about what the word *nurse* means to me.

To me, a nurse:

- takes care of people.
- is highly educated, whether through experience or formal education.
- cares about others.
- is an angel in disguise.
- is strong and independent, and makes quick decisions.
- is a team player.
- is positive.
- is hopeful.
- believes in miracles.
- understands that some things just can't be explained.
- knows that all you can do is your best.
- hopes for the best, prepares for the worst.
- is organized.
- can prioritize.
- can assess a situation immediately.
- can tell when something isn't right.

- is quick to stick up for her patient.
- can stand up to anyone who isn't doing what's best for her patient.
- can start IVs with her eyes closed.
- can say a thousand words with a touch.
- knows just the right thing to say and when to say it.
- has lots of allies.
- speaks up for those who can't speak for themselves.
- has an iron bladder—can hold her pee for countless hours.
- can go all day without eating.
- can find anything.
- can fix any broken IV pole or bedrail without tools.
- can make the TV work.
- knows the magic for getting the computer to turn back on without IT.
- can't remember a password she has had for years, but knows all her patients' names.
- can write a five-hundred-page note quicker than she can fill five spaces in on the computer.
- can't remember which side of the hallway the odd-room numbers are.
- can tell you the last time each of her patients was medicated and with what.
- has at least forty-five doctors' phone numbers memorized.
- has found an empty room to cry in so no one can see.
- can make a bed in less than two minutes.
- can go from crying with one patient to laughing with the next in less than two minutes.
- has a heart of gold.

- has the courage of a tiger.
- has the loyalty of a saint.
- has the strength of ten.
- has a high pain tolerance.
- has a high patience tolerance.
- can hold down a screaming three-year-old child.
- has a heart three sizes too big.
- can cry when she needs to and hide it when she needs to.
- can work until the work is done.
- always has her coworkers' backs.
- always has her patients' backs.
- will respect the wishes of her patient.
- knows where to find anything.
- can figure it out.
- will find out the answer.
- knows the best shoes to wear.
- has all of her pockets full.
- has at least three medication tops in one of her pockets.
- can get what you need if she doesn't have it in her pockets.
- could retire if you paid her $1 for every pen she can produce from her locker, purse, or home, but has none in her pocket
- only has black pens—don't ask her for a blue one.
- can't remember where she left her computer but knows the room numbers of all her patients.
- knows which rooms have the best views.
- knows which rooms are the warmest or coldest.
- knows where an extra pillow is.

- believes in warm blankets.
- lights up the whole room when she smiles.
- knows that a cool washcloth makes everything better.
- can live on nothing but coffee for days.
- knows everyone's official signature by sight.
- can fix the call light.
- knows just when to stick her head in and check on her patient.
- has a stethoscope that fits only her neck.
- has at least four alcohol pads in her pocket.
- always wears her name badge, but it never faces forward.
- hides her angel wings well.
- hides her "don't mess with my patient" horns well.
- can hold a four-hundred-pound confused patient down with one hand.
- gives the best hugs.
- knows when to listen.
- knows when to talk.
- knows just when you need a hug.
- knows where the extra wheelchair is hidden.
- has enough gum for all her coworkers.
- has the best smile.
- has the biggest tears.
- knows how to hide what she's really thinking or feeling.
- can eat, chart, organize, and talk all at the same time.
- can feel a heart rate for four seconds and tell you the rate.
- can look at a patient and tell you their O2 saturation.

- can touch a diabetic patient's arm and tell you the blood glucose.
- knows what's wrong with the patient before they even call the doctor.
- wears a stethoscope and knows how to use it, but doesn't always need it.
- can rock a small child to sleep.
- can hold the hand of a dying man and smile.
- can give you a shot before you even know you've had it.
- can talk you into anything.
- knows when to talk.
- knows when to be quiet.
- thinks about some of her patients long after she has left the hospital.
- feels like no matter what she does, it isn't enough.
- is torn between taking care of her patients and her family.
- can make it down the hall in under two seconds, no matter her age.
- always understands.
- knows just the right tone to use with a patient—whether it's a crying child, a frustrated family member, a scared patient, or someone who just needs to be mad.
- knows how to play her cards.
- like Kenny Rogers, knows when to hold, when to fold, when to walk away, and when to run.
- deserves more money but would never walk out on a hospital full of patients because she can't get a raise.
- always has a smile for anyone who needs it.

- knows when a soft touch is needed.
- knows when a firm touch is needed.
- knows when to just sit quietly with the patient.
- can catch and restrain a three-hundred-pound man before he even realizes he was going down.
- exists on some form of caffeine.
- hates white uniforms and nursing caps.
- loves seeing big veins on people's arms.
- has been known to ask if she can "feel your veins" even in public.
- can hold five times her weight, and more, if she needs to.
- can chart, listen to the call light, knows who's at the nursing station, check her phone for messages from her kids, and know the time (without looking at a clock)—all simultaneously.
- only considers it multitasking if its more than five things at once—the rest is just what she does.
- always thinks that tomorrow will be better.
- almost never calls into work.
- should be taken to the ER *if she ever does* call into work—because that means it's bad enough she needs to be admitted.

About the Author

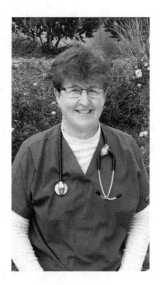

I was born in the very small town of Mayo as a second child to a family with a love of children. We had a farm, and to say that I had an ideal childhood would be putting it mildly. I was taught to work hard and to play hard, with a love for family and friends.

Besides my brother as a playmate, my life was filled with a variety of friends, as well as animals: horses, cows, chickens, pigs, dogs, cats, and everything else that was on Old McDonald's farm.

My dream of being a vet was obvious, but the dedication of going to school for that long was not there. Summer jobs as a nurse's aide led me to a life as a nurse.

My one and only true love is my daughter, Megan, who is married, and I am eagerly awaiting the title of Grandma.

My hobbies include fishing, fishing, and fishing. I don't care what kind, and I don't even care if I catch anything. I just love being at the water on a beautiful day. I enjoy golf and pretty much anything outdoors, whether I'm good at it or not.

I have worked my entire RN career at Tallahassee Memorial Healthcare and I have retired at least three times, but my love for what I do keeps bringing me back, back to nursing and back to the same hospital that has been so supportive of me throughout my career.

I discovered my love for writing during one of my short retirement phases and have enjoyed writing in a variety of different genres.

My Blue Heeler, Kitt Katt, keeps me occupied when I'm not at work, and she loves to fish as much as I do.

My mama and brother still live on the farm I grew up on, and it will always be home. You can take the girl out of the country, but you can never take the country out of the girl.

REFERENCES

Notes

[1] Levine, Irwin, and L. Russell Brown. "Tie a Yellow Ribbon Round the Ole Oak Tree." *Tie a Yellow Ribbon*. Bell Records, 1973.

[2] Badham, John, dir. *WarGames*. Metro-Goldwyn-Mayer Studios, 1983.

[3] Dyer, Frank Lewis, and Thomas Commerford Martin. *Edison: His Life and Inventions*. Vol. 2. Harper & Brothers, 1910, p. 615–616.

[4] Hand, David, dir. *Bambi*. Walt Disney Productions, 1942.

CPSIA information can be obtained
at www.ICGtesting.com
Printed in the USA
LVHW051156220722
724085LV00006B/818